American
Medical
Education

AMERICAN MEDICAL EDUCATION

The Formative Years,

1765-1910

MARTIN KAUFMAN

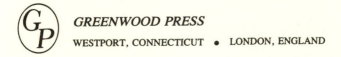

GREENWOOD PRESS

WESTPORT, CONNECTICUT ● LONDON, ENGLAND

Library of Congress Cataloging in Publication Data

Kaufman, Martin, 1941-
    American medical education.

    Bibliography: p.
    Includes index.
    1. Medical education—United States—History.
I. Title [DNLM: 1. History of medicine, modern—United States.
2. Education, medical—History—United States. W18 K21a]
R745.K36   610'.7'1173   75-35346
ISBN 0-8371-8590-4

Library of Congress Catalog Card Number: 75-35346
ISBN: 0-8371-8590-4

First published in 1976

Greenwood Press, a division of Williamhouse-Regency Inc.
51 Riverside Avenue, Westport, Connecticut 06880

Printed in the United States of America

To Dr. John Duffy,
Teacher, scholar, and friend

Contents

Preface

In the course of my research on the history of homeopathy in America, I became aware of the need for a greater understanding of the development of modern medical education. Yet when the historian searches for scholarly works on the history of medical education, he is likely to be disappointed. There are many histories of individual medical schools, most of which are written as if that school was the only one, or the best one. Except for the pioneering work of William Frederick Norwood on the period before the Civil War, there are no books and only a handful of articles that attempt to explain developments in historical perspective.

This book is an attempt to fill the need for synthesis in the field. Yet it is not a history of American medical education. Neither is it a history of the various medical schools. Rather, it is an examination of the major trends and developments that affected the colleges. This book is written in the hope that it will help others to understand how changes in medical education were related to the social and cultural milieu, to scientific developments, and to problems within the medical profession itself.

I have been blessed with a great deal of cooperation from medical historians, librarians, colleagues, friends, and family. I am most indebted to Dr. John Duffy of the University of Maryland. Dr. Duffy not only read the entire manuscript and made valuable suggestions, but as my major professor at Pittsburgh and Tulane, he was responsible for developing my interest in the history of medicine.

Dr. Edward C. Atwater of the University of Rochester School of Medicine provided me with a copy of his paper on the Rochester medical profession, and Dr. Leslie Hanawalt of Wayne State University sent a great deal of material on the Detroit Medical College and

ix

offered suggestions for locating material on the Association of American Medical Colleges. Elizabeth Thomson of Yale University provided information on the early history of Yale's medical school, along with a carefully annotated copy of her article on Thomas Bond.

A number of librarians and archivists provided valuable assistance in locating material and providing needed information. Among these were Manfred Waserman of the National Library of Medicine, Warren Albert of the Archives of the American Medical Association, Roy P. Basler of the Library of Congress, Richard Wolfe of the Countway Library of Harvard University, and William K. Beatty of the Church Medical Library of Northwestern University. The author is indebted to the staffs of the Boston Public Library, the Archives of Medical History at the University of Cincinnati, the Columbia University Library, the Detroit Public Library, the Massachusetts Historical Society, the New York Academy of Medicine, the New York Public Library, and the Library of the University of Vermont.

One friend and colleague at Westfield State College deserves mention. Dr. Robert T. Brown, chairman of the history department, helped to create an atmosphere conducive to scholarship, research, and writing.

Finally I must express my deep appreciation to my wife Henrietta, whose assistance, encouragement, and understanding were crucial for the successful completion of this book.

American
Medical
Education

1
The Colonial
Background

When the first European colonists landed in the New World, one of the earliest problems facing them was that of illness and disease. Take Virginia as an example of the magnitude of the problem. From the time of the first arrival in Jamestown to May 1618, 1,800 persons left England for Virginia. Of these, approximately 100 returned to England and another 1,100 died either in passage or in the colony itself. When a census was taken at the end of 1618, only 600 persons were in Virginia. From 1619 to 1625 another 4,749 immigrants arrived in the colony, but in 1625 the total population of Virginia was only 1,025. Sickness and disease had decimated the population. Similar statistics exist for the Plymouth colony in Massachusetts.[1]

The early settlers had to endure primitive living conditions and inadequate food and water supplies. Epidemic disease periodically swept through the villages, wreaking havoc among those who had left England to find a better life in the New World. To make matters worse, very few trained physicians migrated to the colonies.

It is commonly said that "dukes do not emigrate." Those who came to America tended to be misfits in one way or another. Some were misfits in a religious sense: men and women whose ideas differed from those of the established churches or whose practices and beliefs led to their persecution by the orthodox religions. Others were

3

misfits in an economic sense: they were failures who left Europe in the hope of being more successful three thousand miles from home. Still others were social misfits: in some cases criminals were sentenced to life in America. That was an ideal way to reduce England's increasing crime rate, by sending the criminals to a wilderness across the Atlantic. Political dissenters joined those who came for religious, economic, or social reasons, in a movement away from the stifling European atmosphere and to a more promising future in the New World.

Emigration to the New World meant undergoing a long and dangerous ocean voyage, facing new problems in a strange new land, and accepting what might be a lifelong separation from family and friends. All immigrants were gambling that the future would be better than the past. This being the case, very few successful physicians had the need or the desire to leave Europe.

Yet medical care was a necessity. The companies that established colonies to provide financial gain for investors, such as the London Company at Jamestown or the Dutch West India Company at New Amsterdam, tended to the medical needs of their settlers by sending surgeons or apothecaries to serve for specific periods of time. The Dutch sent men known as "comforters of the sick," and surgeons are reported to have landed with the Dutch colonists. Very little is known about the training of these men, but it is likely that had they been successful practitioners in Europe they never would have agreed to provide medical care for the colonists. Some might have been trained at the medical school at Leyden, however, and those few would have been fairly well-qualified physicians.[2]

In 1628 the Massachusetts Bay Company dispatched two physicians to provide medical care in the colony, and the following year Lambert Wilson, a "chirurgeon," was sent for a period of three years, not only to cure the sick, but also to "educate and instruct in his art one or more youths."[3]

When Puritan congregations followed the lead of their ministers and set out to establish a wilderness Zion in the New World, they undoubtedly included any physicians who were members of the congregation. These men who came for religious reasons may have had an adequate medical training.

Generally, however, those physicians who came to settle in the

colonies were poorly trained and unsuccessful in their medical practices at home. Nathan Smith Davis, who played a major role in the
nineteenth-century drive to reform medical education, stated in his
History of Medical Education that only those "who failed to obtain a
practice at home, or were too conscious of their own unfitness to
make the attempt, emigrated to America."[4]

Many of the factors that discouraged physicians from coming to
America played significant roles in preventing the improvement of
the quality of American medical practice in the early years. For
instance, the expense and danger of the ocean voyage, which certainly convinced a great many to remain in Europe and make the best
of their situation, made it difficult for young Americans to attend
European medical schools in large numbers. On the other hand,
factors that impelled people to leave Europe for America played a
similar role. The Puritan rejection of the Church of England, which
led directly to the establishment of the Massachusetts Bay Colony,
prevented fathers from letting their sons seek a medical education in
England where their religious ideals might be tainted by contact with
the Anglicans, who controlled England's colleges.

Yet there were a great many contacts between the colonies and the
mother country. Although "the Atlantic posed special problems of
communication," there certainly was "a transatlantic community in
the seventeenth century, maintained through a network of relation-
ships between London and Boston, London and New York, and
London and Virginia." The network was composed of people, books,
and ideas. "Officials, clergy, and merchants traveled back and forth
across the ocean," and in addition there was a "transatlantic commercial web which provided the requisite information, credit, and capital
for goods to flow at a profit."[5] But the fact remains that the colonies
had a shortage of physicians who were trained in Europe.

In the absence of sufficient physicians, others assumed medical
leadership. In Puritan New England, clergymen, being the best
educated and most highly respected citizens, provided medical
advice as well as religious and moral assistance. Cotton Mather, the
leading minister of his time, wrote medical works and played a
prominent role in the introduction of inoculation against smallpox.
He even participated in the autopsy of one of his sons. The minister-
physician was also common in England during the seventeenth cen-

tury, indicative of the relation between early American and English culture. During the period of the Great Awakening, from the 1720s to the 1740s, the revival of religious fervor led to a corresponding return of the minister-physician. Jonathan Edwards, the leading light of the movement in the Connecticut River Valley, gave medical as well as theological advice. In one letter he suggested that it would be best "to throw by the doctors and be your own Physician" and recommended a concoction prepared from "one Rattle-Snake," as well as from ginseng.[6]

By and large, however, the medical needs of the colonists were in the hands of poorly educated men who had learned their profession through apprenticeship. Often their preceptor, the physician under whom they studied and learned, was similarly educated by apprenticeship. As the years passed, it seems that the medical situation was getting worse. Death was removing those few trained physicians who had arrived with the early settlers, and by 1700 their places were being taken by local youths who learned from their preceptors rather than through formal education at the universities of Europe.

Training by apprenticeship was fully in line with the European example, especially for surgeons and apothecaries. In order to be considered as a "physician," however, the student had to graduate from a university. A father with the necessary means would apprentice his sons to a craftsman who would agree to teach them his trade, in exchange for a sum of money and the labor of the youth. It was strictly a business deal, with legal indenture papers being signed, describing the obligations of physician and student. The terms of the indenture were normally stringent. The apprentice would be sworn to absolute obedience to his master, promise not to marry, play cards or dice, and agree "not to frequent taverns, alehouses or playhouses."[7]

After the term of apprenticeship had ended, the young man would be certified by the craftsman as being fully qualified to practice the trade, and the student would set out on his own as an independent businessman. In 1786, for instance, John Noyes of Lyme, Connecticut, certified that his apprentice, Richard Ely of Saybrook, "hath been liberally educated and been a student with me in the theory and practice of medicine and surgery, and whereas, said Ely hath made great improvement in the art of physic and surgery, he is well qualified for a practitioner in said arts." Noyes' certificate concluded with the statement that he recommended Ely "as a safe, judicious and able physician, and well qualified to practice."[8]

Because medicine was considered to be no different from any other trade, medical apprenticeship was similar to that of blacksmithing, coopering, or printing.[9] The term of apprenticeship for medical training in colonial America was generally from five to seven years. As in other trades, boys were bound to their masters at relatively young ages. At fourteen or fifteen, John Bard became apprenticed to John Kearsley of Philadelphia; at fifteen, Benjamin Rush was bound to John Redman for a six-year term; and at seventeen, James Lloyd was apprenticed to a Dr. Clark of Boston for a five-year term.[10]

The physician would allow the student to "read medicine" in his library, and he would take his apprentice on his rounds. The boy would learn by watching his master attend to patients and by reading the medical books in his master's library. The apprentice acted as a body servant to the physician, caring for his horse, sweeping the office, and often being sent out to try to collect fees. Undoubtedly bill collecting (and the problems encountered) was an education in itself, possibly discouraging the budding Hippocrates of the eighteenth century.

If the preceptor were well trained and university educated and if he had a genuine interest in elevating the medical practice of the region, the results of this system were laudable. On the other hand, since most colonial practitioners were poorly educated products of the apprenticeship system, it can be assumed that for most apprentices medical training was sketchy at best—reading in a limited library and being taught by a practitioner who had little knowledge to impart. The result, of course, was to perpetuate the conditions; the new generation of physicians would be inadequately trained.

There is ample evidence of the benefits of apprenticeship to the university-trained physician. For instance, Alexander Hamilton and Gustavus Brown, both of Maryland, produced well-educated apprentices who were to serve the region well as medical doctors for many years to come. Yet it certainly can be expected that Daniel Drake's experience was more typical, considering the fact that so few practitioners were well-enough educated to provide anything but rudimentary training for their apprentices. In 1800 at the age of sixteen, Drake began his medical study as apprentice to William Goforth, who himself had been trained by a preceptor. Goforth had a small library, which apparently did not include the leading medical works of the day, such as Cullen's *Materia Medica* and Haller's *Physiology*. Drake was set to work memorizing texts; Goforth had no specimens, plates, or skeletons to provide illustrations for his student. It is unlikely that Drake dissected as part of his training. Basically he served as a body servant; he fed, watered, and saddled the horse, swept the shop, and delivered medicine.[11]

By the start of the eighteenth century, the early colonial period had clearly ended. With it disappeared the "starving time" the first arrivals had faced. The colonies were prosperous and the conditions were now more appealing to the upper classes of Europe. By 1700 medical graduates were more likely to migrate, and migrate they did.[12]

European physicians seemed to flock to the colonies. One historian, Wyndham Blanton, made an extensive survey of foreign-born physicians who settled in Virginia during the eighteenth century, and he found that twenty-three were from Scotland, eleven from England, four from France, two from Switzerland, one from either Portugal or Italy, one from Germany, and one from Italy. Many others came to other colonies. They included men who were soon to be the most eminent of the colonial medical profession, simply by virtue of the fact that they were the only university-educated physicians in America. To New York came Cadwalader Colden, Samuel Clossy, and Peter Middleton. To Maryland came Gustavus Brown and Charles F. Wiesenthal. South Carolina became the home of Lionel Chalmers, John Lining, and Alexander Garden. William Hunter arrived in Newport, Rhode Island, in 1752. William Douglass was an early arrival to Boston in 1713, and at that time he was the only university-educated physician in the city. To Pennsylvania came John Kearsley, who became the preceptor to some of Philadelphia's most eminent physicians, including William Shippen, and John Bard, whose sons were to be pioneers in the founding of the first two medical schools in America. In addition Kearsley was master to John Redman, who became preceptor to John Morgan, Benjamin Rush, and Caspar Wistar, all of whom became prominent physicians and professors in the first medical school in America.[13]

These late arrivals to the American scene revolutionized medical practice by instilling in their students a desire for more than a rudimentary medical training. Benjamin Rush's *Memorial* of his student days gives a fine impression of the value of these excellent and dedicated preceptors. In February 1761 Rush began the study of medicine as apprentice to John Redman. In more than five years, Rush "was absent from his business but eleven days, and never spent more than three evenings out of his house." Redman had the most extensive clientele of any Philadelphia physician, and "as he had at no time more than two apprentices, he kept them constantly employed. In addition to preparing and compounding medicines, visiting the sick and performing many little offices of a nurse to them," Rush took "exclusive charge" of Redman's books and accounts. "I read in the intervals of business and at late and early hours all the books in medicine that were put into my hands by my master," Rush said, "or that I could borrow from other students of medicine in the city. I studied Dr. Boerhaave's lectures upon physiology and pathology with the closest attention, and abridged a considerable part of Van Swieten's commentaries upon his practical aphorisms. I kept a common place book in which I recorded everything that I thought curious or valuable in my reading and in my master's practice." Redman instilled in Rush an "estimation" for the ideas of Sydenham, "frequently alluding to his opinions and practice, particularly in the treatment of epidemics." In addition, because Redman was physician to the Pennsylvania Hospital, Rush "was admitted to see the practice of five other physicians besides his own in the hospital."[14]

It is obvious that the caliber of training received at the hands of men like John Redman was far superior to that provided by less dedicated men who themselves were trained through apprenticeship. Indeed, upon completing their apprenticeship, their students often boarded ship for Europe, where they completed their education at leading universities. Early in the century, Americans enrolled at Leyden where they came under the influence of the great clinical teacher, Boerhaave. By the middle of the century, however, Edinburgh, with William Cullen and Alexander Monro on the faculty, had become much more popular than Leyden for American students. Before 1776 forty-one Americans attended Edinburgh; by 1812 there were 139 American graduates.[15]

When they had completed their formal education, having been awarded their M.D. degrees, American students normally spent some time traveling in England and on the Continent. They walked the wards of Guy's Hospital or St. Thomas's in London, or L'Hôtel Dieu in Paris, taking advantage of the abundant clinical resources. There they learned through observation about the treatment of unfamiliar diseases. They enrolled in the anatomy classes established by John and William Hunter or the obstetrics classes of Colin McKenzie. They studied with William Cheselden, the London surgeon, and they attended William Smellie's lectures on midwifery. Their thirst for knowledge carried them to the leading European physicians and surgeons.[16]

Their thirst, however, did not stop with medical matters. Being from upper-class families, the American students in Europe managed to attend numerous parties and balls, moving in the upper crust of European society. In some cases, their social activities forced them to move on to other European centers of medical training. Such was the case with Thomas Ruston, a student at Edinburgh in 1764. In a letter to his father, Ruston described an episode that nearly forced him into matrimony. He met a "Laidy, worth about £500 Sterling," with "the best of Connexions, being a branch of Lord Montroses family." After he had seen the young lady a number of times, the conversation turned to America. Ruston suggested that she go there, and after consulting with friends and relatives, she agreed. "Not many days after," according to Ruston, "some Laidies began to *wish me Joy, they Congratulated me on the Choice I had made, & wisht us a great deal of happiness &c., &c."* Ruston was shocked to learn that his friendly conversation had been taken as a proposal of marriage. He severed the connection with a show of "indifference" to her, and with a story of changed plans in which he would go to Holland, France, and then London, he escaped the young lady's clutches.[17]

Unfortunately, only a small percentage of the American physicians completed their education in Europe. From 1607 to 1776 more than 3,000 physicians practiced in America; of that number, fewer than 400 had received medical degrees, mostly in Europe.[18] The vast majority of America's physicians either were trained by apprenticeship or were mere pretenders, men who "suddenly" decided to abandon other pursuits in favor of medical practice. Among the latter was a fellow in Huntington, Long Island, who was described in 1744 by Dr. Alexander Hamilton. Hamilton discovered that he "had been a shoemaker in town and was a notable fellow at his trade, but happening two years agoe to cure an old woman of a pestilent mortall disease, he thereby acquired the character of a physitian, was applied to from all quarters, and finding the practice of physick a more profitable business than cobling, he laid aside his awls and leather, got himself some gallipots, and instead of cobling of soals, fell to cobling of human bodies."[19]

The cobbler who transformed himself into a practicing physician might have been typical of the situation within the medical profession, if one can judge from reports in colonial newspapers. For instance, in 1753 the *Independent Reflector,* a New York City journal, commented on the "dismal Havock made by Quacks and Pretenders." The editor noted that New York City had more than forty physicians, but most were "meer pretenders" who were "Ignorant as Boys of the lowest Class in a Reading-School." When spoken to, these physicians soon betrayed "their natural Stupidity and Ignorance!" The editor called them "licensed Assassins" and rhetorically asked, "How many of the Lives of the good people of this City must annually fall a Sacrifice to those Pests of Society, those merciless Butchers of Human Kind!" He concluded by replying: "The Blood of my Countrymen calls for Vengeance upon the Wretches that Lavish it like water, and afterwards fall upon the bereaved Widow and Orphan, with an extortionate Bill."[20]

In 1766 the *New-York Mercury* published an article on the abuses perpetrated by the so-called physicians of the city. It charged they stole twenty thousand pounds from "the purses of the Publick, under the specious pretense of acting the physician." That was "an enormous sum to murder mankind." To the author, the one hundred quacks in the city were "plagues extraordinary," while the "diseases which Nature already affords are numerous enough." The article concluded with a plea for the passage of laws to prevent medical quackery.[21]

Later that year, a letter to the *Boston Gazette* echoed the words of the *Mercury.* Noting that "pretended doctors have slain their thousands; but happily for them the ground covers their miscarriages," the author expressed a wish that the competent physicians would do something to "at least prevent the infection from spreading any farther." He blamed the condition on the inadequate medical education of the day. No physician would accept an apprentice, the author declared, unless he had from eighty to one hundred pounds. "Practitioners instead of endeavoring to instill into their pupils a due respect for the health of their fellow-creatures, consider them only as they do their patients, from whom they expect to receive handsome fees."[22]

In 1785 a letter to the editor of the *Maryland Journal and Baltimore Advertiser* expressed similar sentiments. The writer complained about the men who "daily intrude themselves upon the public, as proficients in the healing art, totally unqualified for their important task." The sick person reaches out for help, but instead of help he often received "a deadly potion, proffered with merely a prospect of reward." The "highwayman may be satisfied with your purse," the writer exclaimed, "while the obdurate heart of the quack, insensible to every finer sensation, continues to thirst after lucre, even at the expense of your life." He concluded with a plea for a medical license law that would allow a group of responsible and competent physicians to examine all those wishing to become medical doctors.[23]

Obviously there was a desperate need to eliminate the chaos that had developed in the medical profession. By the 1760s, the desire for reform was clearly evident among a number of leading physicians. The Seven Years' War apparently played a major role in convincing members of the medical profession of their inadequate training. Many Americans served as assistant regimental surgeons, and their contact with better-trained British military surgeons forced them to recognize their own insufficient educational background.[24] William F. Norwood, a pioneer historian of American medical education, has suggested that the recognition of their "academic deficiencies" encouraged the colonial physicians to work for the passage of medical license legislation and to develop medical societies, the first steps toward true professionalization.[25]

As early as 1735, William Douglass helped to found a medical society in Boston, and others were established in Litchfield County, Connecticut, and in New Jersey in 1766. The proceedings of the New Jersey medical society in its early years indicates intense interest in improving medical education. In fact, at its May 5, 1767, meeting it was decided to try to solve the problem once and for all. After some discussion the members agreed "for the advantage of youth and the honor of the art, that no student be hereafter taken an apprentice by any member, unless he has a competent knowledge of the Latin and some initiation in the Greek." (As shall be seen, one of the leading areas of reform in later years was foreshadowed by the New Jersey society with its early demand for preliminary education of medical students.) They also agreed that no member of the society should take an apprentice for a period of fewer than four years, three of which should be "spent with his master," with the fourth "in some medical college in America or Europe."[26] This was an early realization of the need for formal medical education to supplement the training received from the preceptor.

In 1760 the first law regulating the practice of medicine was passed; it was effective only in New York City. The preamble to the act explained the need for its passage: "Whereas many ignorant and unskilful persons in Physic and Surgery, in order to gain a subsistence, do take upon themselves to administer physic, and to practice surgery, in the city of New York, to the endangering the lives and limbs of their patients; and many poor and ignorant people inhabiting the said city, who have been persuaded to become their patients, have been great sufferers thereby;—for preventing such abuses in future." The law provided that every student undergo an examination by the members of His Majesty's Council and physicians selected to assist them.[27] In 1772 New Jersey followed with a similar law. By 1815 societies had been established in most of the states, and these organizations worked diligently for the passage of medical license legislation. By the 1830s, according to Nathan S. Davis, only three states lacked such laws.[28]

Among the earliest steps toward the formal education of physicians were the demonstrations and anatomical lectures given by several physicians for the benefit of medical students and other interested citizens. In 1730 Thomas Cadwalader, who had learned anatomy under the British surgeon William Cheselden, gave a series of demonstrations, as he again did from 1745 to 1751. John Bard and Peter Middleton dissected the human body for the instruction of students in New York City in 1750. From 1754 through 1756 William Hunter, a young Scottish physician, gave a similar demonstration and lectured at Newport, Rhode Island.[29] Hunter's lectures were apparently "old Dr. Monro's lectures, as far as regarded the order and the physiological and pathological remarks," but the significance was not in the content of the lectures themselves but in the fact that formal lectures were being presented, which could only benefit the citizenry by providing additional education to the physicians and students who attended.[30] (Incidentally, in a letter describing the work of Hunter, Benjamin Waterhouse commented on the fact that Hunter not only taught anatomy but produced it. His daughter was *"the fairest among the fair."* "Such a piece of anatomy and physiology mine eyes never beheld," exclaimed the Boston physician.)[31]

The first substantial step toward a true reform of medical education came with the establishment of formal medical colleges, which were natural extensions of the earlier anatomy demonstrations. Schools enabled students who had served their apprenticeship to attend classes where they would get a rapid review of the branches of medical science, "concentrated into as small a part of the year as possible." The colleges were intended to supplement the work of the preceptor, who might be an excellent practitioner but who was unlikely to have been an expert in all the fields of medicine. In effect, by combining several preceptors into a medical faculty, the student could complete his review in a period of five or six months. The students studied anatomy by dissection and chemistry by laboratory experiments, and they clinically observed a wide variety of patients at a local hospital. All these were not at all practical in the preceptor's office.[32]

At a time when medical knowledge was definitely limited, it was not unreasonable that in a short period students could benefit from a rapid review of anatomy, physiology, materia medica (classification and description of treatments), therapeutics, obstetrics, and chemistry. After all, to a very large extent, the principal works were limited to medical practice by Sydenham, Boerhaave, and Cullen; physiology by Haller; anatomy by Cheselden and Monro; surgery by Pott, Sharp, and Jones; midwifery by Hunter and Smellie; materia medica by Lewis.[33]

With this in mind, the first medical colleges were established in the colonies. These schools provided a great service to the profession by enabling more physicians to receive the training that previously was restricted to those who could afford to spend years in Europe. Now, after an apprenticeship with a country practitioner, the student would be able to enroll in a medical college, complete the review, and enter practice far better qualified than if he had just come from the office of his preceptor.

Notes

1. John Duffy, *Epidemics in Colonial America* (Baton Rouge, 1953), pp. 12-13. See also John Blake, "Diseases and Medical Practice in Colonial America," *International Record of Medicine* 171 (June 1958): 350-351.

2. Genevieve Miller, "Medical Education in the American Colonies," *Journal of Medical Education* 31 (February 1956): 83ff.; Claude Heaton, "Medicine in New York During the English Colonial Period," *Bulletin of the History of Medicine* 17 (January 1945): 9-37; and William D. Postell, "Medical Education and Medical Schools in Colonial America," *International Record of Medicine* 171 (June 1958): 364.

3. Massachusetts Bay Company to Endicott, April 17, 1629, quoted in *Boston Medical and Surgical Journal* 106 (April 13, 1882): 341-342.

4. N. S. Davis, *History of Medical Education and Institutions in the United States, from the First Settlement of the British Colonies to the Year 1850* (Chicago, 1851), p. 18.

5. Lawrence A. Cremin, *American Education: The Colonial Experience* (New York, 1970), pp. 232-235. See also Bernard Bailyn, *Education in the Forming of American Society* (Chapel Hill, 1960), and Bernard Bailyn, "Communications and Trade: The Atlantic in the Seventeenth Century," *Journal of Economic History* 13 (1953): 378-387.

6. See Otho T. Beall and Richard H. Shryock, *Cotton Mather: First Significant Figure in American Medicine* (Baltimore, 1954): Jonathan Edwards to Mrs. Esther Burr, Stockbridge, Mass., March 28, 1753, Boston Public Library.

7. Wyndham Blanton, *Medicine in Virginia in the 17th Century* (Richmond, 1930), p. 76.

8. Quoted in Herbert Thoms, *Jared Eliot* (n.p., 1967), p. 23.

9. Genevieve Miller, "Medical Apprenticeship in the American Colonies," *Ciba Symposia* 8 (January 1947): 502-510.

10. Joseph M. Toner, *Contributions to the Annals of Medical Progress and Medical Education in the United States Before and During the War of Independence* (Washington, D.C., 1874), p. 104.

11. Emmet Field Horine, *Daniel Drake* (Philadelphia, 1961), pp. 74ff. See also Toner, *Contributions to the Annals of Medical Progress,* p. 104.

12. This point is well taken by Genevieve Miller, "European Influences in Colonial Medicine," *Ciba Symposia* 8 (January 1947): 512-513. For a composite view of the colonial practitioners, see Whitfield J. Bell, Jr., "A Portrait of the Colonial Physician," *Bulletin of the History of Medicine* 44 (November-December 1970): 497-517.

13. Quoted in Miller, "European Influences in Colonial Medicine," 513-15.

14. Benjamin Rush, *A Memorial Containing Travels Through Life or Sundry Incidents in the Life of Dr. Benjamin Rush,* quoted in Miller, "Medical Education in the American Colonies," 87-88.

15. Miller, "European Influences in Colonial Medicine," 518; Miller, "Medical Education in the American Colonies," 89-90.

16. The specifics of the Edinburgh education are described by Whitfield J. Bell, Jr., "Medical Students and Their Examiners in Eighteenth Century America," *Transactions and Studies of the College of Physicians of Philadelphia,* 4th ser. 21 (June 1953): 14-24. See also Miller, "Medical Education in the American Colonies," 89. The description of Rush's European education in Nathan S. Goodman, *Benjamin Rush: Physician and Citizen* (Philadelphia, 1934), pp. 8-19 should be seen, along with Carl Binger, *Revolutionary Doctor* (New York, 1966). A brief description of education is given in John Cary, *Joseph Warren: Physician, Politican, Patriot* (Urbana, Illinois, 1961), pp. 16-17.

17. Thomas Ruston to Job Ruston, Edinburgh, September 30, 1769, Ruston Papers, Library of Congress.

18. N. S. Davis, *Contributions to the History of Medical Education and Medical Institutions in the United States of America, 1776-1876* (Washington, D.C., 1877), p. 9.

19. Alexander Hamilton, *Gentleman's Progress: The Itineratum of Dr. Alexander Hamilton, 1744* (Chapel Hill, 1948), quoted in Blake, "Diseases and Medical Practice in Colonial America," 359.

20. *Independent Reflector* (New York City), February 15, 1753.

21. *New-York Mercury,* October 13, 1766.

22. *Boston Gazette,* December 15, 1766.

23. *Maryland Journal and Baltimore Advertiser,* December 13, 1785. For similar quotations from eighteenth-century physicians and observers, see Blake, "Diseases and Medical Practice in Colonial America," 358ff.

24. Brooke Hindle, *The Pursuit of Science in Revolutionary America* (Chapel Hill, 1956), pp. 110ff.

25. William F. Norwood, "The Mainstream of American Medical Education, 1765-1965," *Annals of the New York Academy of Sciences* 128 (September 27, 1965), p. 464.

26. *Transactions of the Medical Society of New Jersey, 1766-1858* (Newark, 1875), pp. 18-19.

27. *American Journal of the Medical Sciences* 20 (August 1837): 469.

28. For a thorough analysis of medical licensing, see Richard H. Shryock, *Medical Licensing in America* (Baltimore, 1967), chap. 1. See also the narrative of the establishment of the New Jersey Medical Society in *New-York Mercury,* March 2, 1767.

29. Postell, "Medical Education and Medical Schools," 367; Davis, *Contributions to the History of Medical Education,* p. 12.

30. Benjamin Waterhouse to Caspar Wistar, Cambridge, September 22, 1808, in *Medical News* (Philadelphia) 41 (July 15, 1882): 79-80.

31. Ibid.

32. Davis, *Contributions to the History of Medical Education,* pp. 25-26. See also N. S. Davis, *Address on the Progress of Medical Education* (Philadelphia, 1876), p. 11.

33. Davis, *Address on the Progress of Medical Education,* p. 12.

2

The Earliest
Medical Schools

The first medical college in the colonies was established in Philadelphia by William Shippen, Jr., and John Morgan.[1] While Shippen and Morgan were students at Edinburgh, they discussed the need for formal medical training in America, and they made specific plans to establish a school upon their return from Europe. They even decided exactly what they would teach: Shippen would lecture in anatomy and obstetrics; Morgan in theory and practice of medicine; Arthur Lee, who was soon to become Shippen's brother-in-law when Shippen married Ann Lee, would teach medical botany; and Theodorick Bland would teach materia medica.[2]

Morgan and Shippen discussed the project with their London and Edinburgh acquaintances, and they must have been so enthusiastic about the need for a school in the colonies that Dr. John Fothergill of London set out to ensure that the dream would become a reality. When Morgan returned from Edinburgh in 1762 he brought from Fothergill a gift of eighteen drawings and plates that were to provide the basis for anatomical teaching at the Pennsylvania Hospital. In July of that year, Fothergill wrote to James Pemberton, a leading Philadelphian, recommending that Shippen give a course of anatomical lectures. In the letter, he expressed his hope that Shippen and Morgan would "be able to erect a school of Physick amongst you that

18

may draw many students from various parts of America and the West
Indies, and at least furnish them with a better idea of the rudiments
of their profession than they have at present the means of acquiring
on your side of the water."[3]

The correspondence of Thomas Ruston, who was at Edinburgh
with Morgan and Shippen, indicates that the college was not simply a
humanitarian venture. There was a significant personal advantage to
being a professor in the early medical schools. In a letter to his father,
Ruston had noted that it might be difficult to make a living by
practicing medicine in Philadelphia. "We may fall upon some easier
method than by the dry Practice of Physic, for that I'm still afraid will
be but a traid in Philad[a]."[4] Ruston desperately wanted to join the
faculty of Shippen's school. Unfortunately, as he confided to his
father, "Morgan has fixed upon the very Branch on w[ch] I intended to
Lecture," and there was little hope that Morgan would resign, "since
it must have cost him a good deal of pains to prepare himself, & he has
so much need of all the advantage he can make in that way."[5]

Another indication of more mercenary and selfish motives can be
seen from the experiences of Benjamin Rush. When he returned to
Philadelphia from Edinburgh, Rush sought an opening at the College
of Philadelphia to enhance his reputation. He did not have a rich
patron or extensive family connections so he was destined to practice
among the poor of the city unless he could advertise himself as a
professor at the medical school. That would place him far above other
physicians in the area.[6]

In any case, for personal reasons as well as to advance the practice
of medicine in the colonies, the medical college was founded. When
Shippen returned to Philadelphia in 1762, he immediately began a
course on anatomy. He advertised in the *Pennsylvania Gazette* that
the course of lectures would help those "now engaged in the Study of
Physic . . . whose Circumstances and Connections will not admit of
their going abroad" to the anatomy schools of Europe. Shippen was
able to use "some curious ANATOMICAL CASTS AND DRAWINGS (just
arrived in the Carolina)" which Fothergill had sent to the Pennsylvania Hospital.[7]

When Morgan returned to the city, he proposed to the trustees of
the College of Philadelphia that they add a medical branch to the
college. The trustees agreed and appointed him professor of the

theory and practice of medicine. Although Shippen had been lecturing on anatomy since 1762, he was not mentioned in the initial
announcement. By the time the course began, however, Shippen
had been appointed professor of anatomy and surgery. On November 14, 1765, the first American medical college opened its
doors.[8]

The previous day, at the commencement of the College of
Philadelphia, Morgan had detailed his plans for the medical school.
His celebrated address, *A Discourse upon the Institution of Medical
Schools in America,* written while he was traveling in Europe, was
presented to the public on May 30 and 31. He noted that with the
apprenticeship system of education physicians could not "ever become more than servile imitators of others." The practitioner "soon
gets through his little stock of knowledge; he repeats over and over
his round of prescriptions."[9] The result of inadequate medical training was obvious to Morgan. "Great is the havock" that the untrained
physician "spreads on every side, robbing the affectionate husband
of his darling spouse, or rendering the tender wife a helpless
widow;—increasing the number of orphans . . . and laying whole
families desolate. Remorseless foe to mankind! activated by more
than savage cruelty! hold, hold," Morgan pleaded, hold "thy exter-
minating hand."[10]

Morgan described the ideal medical college, which was obviously
copied from the Edinburgh example.[11] He required high standards of
preliminary education. "Young men ought to come well prepared for
the study of Medicine," Morgan declared. They should be well
acquainted with Latin, Greek, mathematics, and natural philosophy.
The young Edinburgh graduate advocated the complete medical
curriculum in the college, including anatomy, materia medica,
botany, chemistry, theory of physic, physiology, pathology, and
practice of medicine.

Finally, Morgan recommended that the trustees consider Shippen
for the professorship in anatomy, for he had been lecturing on
anatomy for the past three years and he thus was more experienced
than anyone else in the city.[12] The trustees shortly appointed Shippen
to that post, giving the school a faculty of two young men who had
recently arrived from Edinburgh.

On May 12, 1767, the trustees of the College of Philadelphia decided that granting the "usual degrees" in physic to deserving students would "greatly encourage the Medical School," "promote emulation among the students, and tend to put the Practice of Physic on a more respectable footing in *America.*" They established requirements for the "Bachelor's Degree in Physic." College graduates would be automatically admitted for instruction. Others would have to prove their proficiency in Latin, mathematics, and natural and experimental philosophy. Every student would be required to have served a sufficient apprenticeship with a reputable practitioner and be able to demonstrate a general knowledge of Pharmacy."[13]

A candidate for a "doctor's Degree in Physic" had to be at least twenty-four years of age, have received a bachelor's degree in physic at least three years before, and write and defend a thesis, which had to be published at his own expense. After announcing their degree requirements, the trustees declared that the school was "intended to Benefit mankind" by improving the practice of medicine and by allowing students to receive their education in the colonies.[14]

On June 21, 1768, America's first medical commencement was held in Philadelphia; ten young men were granted degrees of Bachelor of Physic. They included Benjamin Rush, who after completing his studies in Edinburgh eventually became the leading American physician of the early national period. The significance of the day was not lost. The *Boston Chronicle* declared that that day "may be considered as having given birth to medical honours in America."[15]

The ten students had been taught by Shippen, who lectured on chemistry, materia medica, and the theory and practice of medicine, and by Morgan, who taught anatomy and surgery. In addition the students heard Thomas Bond's clinical lectures at the Pennsylvania Hospital. In 1766 Bond had given an introductory lecture to the medical class on the "utility of clinical instruction" in medical education, an address that has been rated second only to Morgan's *Discourse* "in importance for medical education in 18th century America." In his talk, Bond argued that regardless of the proficiency of the professor, instruction through lectures and readings was insufficient preparation for medical practice. Bedside teaching was crucial; "Infirmaries," Bond insisted, were the "Grand Theatres of Medical Knowledge."[16]

In analyzing the actual instruction at the College of Philadelphia, it is apparent that a two-man faculty with adjunct lectures by a clinician was hardly comparable to Edinburgh. Yet it was a great improvement over the traditional training through apprenticeship. According to Whitfield Bell, Morgan's biographer, the program was "not Morgan's course, but Cullen's—and diluted Cullen at that. Authority and detail were lost in the process by which Cullen's lectures were taken down by Morgan in Edinburgh." In addition, Morgan presented two basic sciences in fewer than forty lectures, and he taught chemistry without proper apparatus.[17]

In 1768 and 1769, however, the college expanded, and that expansion substantially improved the quality of education. Adam Kuhn, a pupil of Linnaeus, the great Swedish botanist, was appointed professor of botany and materia medica. The following year, Benjamin Rush, returning from Edinburgh, was appointed professor of chemistry. By then, America's first medical college was performing a great service to the colonies by enabling American students to get the benefit of advanced training without traveling to Europe.

The second medical school in the colonies, like that in Philadelphia, followed the Edinburgh example,[18] and it was influenced by the planning Shippen and Morgan had done. While Samuel Bard of New York City was a student at Edinburgh, he learned that Shippen and Morgan intended to establish a college in Philadelphia. In a letter to his father, Bard wished that it were in New York City so he could participate in so noble a venture. He asked his father for advice, suggesting that perhaps a similar school could be established in New York. Earlier, when John Bard, Samuel's father, had attempted to convince the authorities of King's College of the need to teach anatomy, he was rebuked with the reply: "We have so many of the Faculty already destroying his Majesty's good subjects, that in the humour people are, they had rather one half were hanged that are allready practicing than breed up a New Swarm in addition to the old."[19] Bard informed his son that there was little hope of gaining a collegiate connection. In addition, the elder Bard noted that New York lacked a large hospital for clinical observation; until such a hospital could be established, any medical education offered in the city would be inadequate.

By 1767 Samuel Bard had brought together a medical faculty in spite of his father's discouraging advice. The elder Bard used his influence to get the governors of the college to appoint them to provide "regular Instruction of Gentlemen in the different Branches of MEDICINE." The faculty consisted of six men, three of them among the leading and most experienced members of the New York medical profession: Samuel Clossy, Peter Middleton, and John Jones. The other three professors were young men who had just returned from colleges in Europe: Samuel Bard, John V. B. Tennent, and James Smith.[20]

Samuel Clossy, professor of anatomy, had received his undergraduate training at Trinity College, Dublin, where he had also been awarded degrees of Bachelor of Medicine and Doctor of Medicine. He had been giving private anatomy lectures in New York City since 1763, and he had published a monograph based on four years of clinical and pathological study.[21] Peter Middleton, professor of physiology and pathology, had received his medical training and degree from St. Andrew's in Scotland, and he had taught anatomy with John Bard in the 1750s. The professor of surgery was John Jones, who had studied with William Hunter and Percival Pott in London and who went on to the universities of Edinburgh and Leyden. He took his medical degree from the University of Rheims in 1751. (In 1775 Jones was to publish the first surgical treatise printed in America, a handbook for the military surgeons of the Revolutionary War.)

These three eminent practitioners were joined by the three newcomers. Samuel Bard, professor of the theory and practice of physic, had received his degree from Edinburgh in 1765. He later wrote America's first textbook on obstetrics, as well as accounts of diphtheria and yellow fever. Smith and Tennent had both received their degrees from Leyden in 1764. Tennent became professor of midwifery, and Smith was appointed professor of chemistry and materia medica.

The opening of the King's College Medical School on November 2, 1767, was a festive occasion. The governor and the Supreme Court justices "in their robes" all walked in the processional, along with the professors and officials of the school. At the college hall, they "were entertained" by Middleton's lecture "on the Antiquity, Progress and Usefulness of the Science of Medicine," which demonstrated Middleton's keen interest in the history of medicine; it was later published.[22]

Byron Stookey, the historian of medical education in colonial New York, argues persuasively that although the Philadelphia school was first to be established, it was not a medical college in the true sense of the term, as least not until 1769 when it had a full complement of professors. Until then, the faculty consisted of two young and relatively inexperienced physicians, Morgan and Shippen. On the other hand, when King's College opened in 1767, it had a superior faculty and was a complete medical school following the Edinburgh tradition.[23]

Regardless of the debate over which was first, on May 3, 1769, barely ten months after the first commencement at Philadelphia, King's College graduated its first class. At the commencement, Samuel Bard delivered a "Discourse on the Duties of a Physician," which included an eloquent appeal for the establishment of a public hospital, both to provide treatment for the poor of the city and to offer ample clinical experience for the students. At the "college dinner" following commencement, Bard audaciously passed around a "subscription paper" asking for donations. Sir Henry Moore, the governor of the province, offered £200, and before the dinner had ended, almost £1,000 had been subscribed. Then, £3,000 was added from the budget of the colony, providing the basis for the New York Hospital.[24]

Now that Philadelphia and New York City had established medical colleges, it was expected that other cities would follow their example. In Boston the drive to improve the education of physicians centered on the formation of the Harvard Medical School. Just prior to the Revolutionary War, Dr. Ezekial Hersey of Hingham bequeathed £1,000 to found a professorship in anatomy and physic at the university. At that time, the Harvard Corporation decided that the sum was insufficient to support the professorship; the money was invested in the hope that eventually there would be enough to endow the professorship.[25]

On May 14, 1780, when the Boston Medical Society met at the Green-Dragon Tavern, John Warren made a detailed proposal for a medical college. He even suggested a three-man faculty: Dr. Danforth would teach materia medica and chemistry, Dr. Rand would lecture on the theory and practice of medicine, and Warren would demonstrate anatomy and surgery. Warren's recommendations ran into swift opposition. Danforth declined to teach without adequate chemical apparatus; Rand rejected the idea with the comment, "Who would want to hear an uninteresting course of lectures on fevers and consumptions?" Since Warren was the only one left in the plan and no one volunteered to join him, he lectured for two years on anatomy and surgery.[26]

In spite of the cool reception to his plan, Warren did not forget his dream of a Boston medical college. On September 26, 1782, he wrote to Benjamin Rush for information on the Philadelphia school. Rush replied with a detailed description of the college and its requirements.[27] Armed with this information, Warren made a formal proposal to the members of the Harvard Corporation, and he convinced them of the need to improve medical education in New England. On November 22, 1782, Harvard established a medical college and appointed Warren professor of anatomy and surgery and Benjamin Waterhouse, who had studied at London and Edinburgh, professor of theory and practice. Aaron Dexter was later selected to teach chemistry and materia medica.[28]

On September 11, 1783, the Harvard Corporation published its plans for the new school, along with its requirements. The announcement began with the comment that medical colleges were "of great utility" for a number of reasons. First, it was an advantage for medical students "to be led into the knowledge of the various parts by actual dissection." Then, a knowledge of materia medica and chemistry "by a course of actual experiments" was "of great consequence to any physician." Finally, it was important for physicians to learn the properties of medicines and to be able to analyze and compound them. In spite of the fact that there was a great depreciation of paper money in the aftermath of the Revolutionary War, making Hersey's original bequest inadequate even after eleven years of investment, the Harvard Corporation decided that since medical education was so important, it would establish such a college.[29]

Harvard agreed to provide a medical library, a set of anatomical preparations, and a proper "theatre." Moreover, the corporation would "apply to the legislature" for a law giving the professors the bodies of executed criminals and suicide cases for dissection. Interestingly, the announcement indicated that all students applying for admission would be accepted, whether or not they were college graduates, as long as they paid their fees. It is apparent that the Harvard Corporation intended the school to be totally self-supporting, beyond the initial allocation for materials. Undergraduates, however, would not be admitted until they had two years' standing in the university.[30]

The three professors of the new Harvard Medical School were formally inaugurated in October 1783 in an impressive ceremony similar to that held previously in New York City. The college buildings were illuminated, and the chapel windows contained lights "disposed in form of letters," in honor of the professors, Warren, Waterhouse, and Dexter. Unfortunately Dexter was unable to reach Cambridge in time to be formally inducted, being delayed by what the newspapers described as "contrary winds."[31] The introductory lectures were delivered on the first Friday in December 1783, and Harvard's first course of medical lectures started two weeks later.[32]

Although the college admitted anyone who could pay the fees, it is clear from all descriptions that standards were high. In order to receive a bachelor's degree in physic, students were required to take two courses of lectures in anatomy, theory and practice of medicine, chemistry, and materia medica, and they must have studied two full years as apprentices to reputable practitioners. After having attended the courses of lectures, those students who did not have a college education had to prove their competence in Latin and in experimental philosophy and mathematics. Then all degree candidates were to be publicly examined by the Harvard professors and any members of the Massachusetts Medical Society who chose to attend. Finally, students were required to defend a thesis in either Latin or English. In order to qualify for a doctor's degree, a Bachelor of Physic who had practiced for seven years had to defend a dissertation in both Latin and English and be examined by the professors.[33]

Peter La Terriere, who received a bachelor's degree in 1789, provided an excellent description of the college and its standards. In his oral examination before the faculty and interested citizens, he had to answer such questions as: "Describe the process of deglutition." "Of what is blood composed?" "What is inflammation?" "Did you ever read Sydenham?" "Describe an amputation below the knee."

"How would you deliver the placenta if it did not deliver spontane-
ously?" Then La Terriere was asked by a fellow "from the seats,"
"What was a sudorific and which was the most efficacious?" He
responded, quite appropriately: "A sudorific is anything that pro-
duces perspiration. The best way to make a man sweat that I know of
is to make him stand up in a place like this on a hot afternoon and
answer questions." At that point in the proceedings, he had to deliver
his thesis and answer any and all questions about it.[34]

In 1789, seven years after the founding of the Harvard Medical
School, an attempt was made to establish a similar school in Baltimore. In that year, two relatively young physicians, Andrew Wiesenthal and George Buchanan, returned from Scotland. Almost
immediately, they announced that Buchanan would teach obstetrics,
and local newspapers carried announcements of Wiesenthal's lectures on anatomy, physiology, pathology, and surgery, as well as
"some lectures on the Gravid Uterus." In addition, Wiesenthal
promised to "accommodate two or three private students in his
House, . . . where they will have peculiar Advantages."[35]

The following year, 1790, a number of Baltimore physicians
decided to expand the lectures of Buchanan and Wiesenthal into a
full-scale medical college. On March 29 it was announced that a new
school had been established, with Wiesenthal teaching anatomy,
Buchanan lecturing on midwifery, Samuel Coale demonstrating
chemistry and materia medica, Lyde Goodwin lecturing on the
theory and practice of surgery, and George Brown lecturing on the
theory and practice of medicine.[36] Although classes were to begin the
following winter, the Baltimore school did not open its doors as
scheduled and there was no medical school in Baltimore until 1807.

In 1797, Nathan Smith, a Harvard graduate who had recently
returned from Edinburgh, helped develop the fourth American
medical school, this one at Dartmouth College. Then, just at the turn
of the century, a fifth college was organized—at Transylvania
University in Kentucky. It did not graduate its first student until
1802, however.

The United States was basically an undeveloped frontier society,
and the European system of medical education was not perfectly
suited to it. It was unrealistic to expect the Edinburgh model to serve
the purposes of a land with inadequate primary and secondary

schools and with severe transportation difficulties. The new system required a supply of top-flight medical professors at a time when very few Americans had had the opportunity to acquire the requisite knowledge and experience. This is obvious from the fact that so many of the professors were young men in their twenties, just out of Edinburgh or Leyden. They had no real opportunity to gain extensive experience, except what they could glean from walking the wards of Europe's hospitals and studying for a short time with Europe's leading specialists. Morgan, Shippen, Rush, Bard, Smith, Wiesenthal, Buchanan, and Lee were all in that category.

The inevitable results were lectures copied verbatim from notes taken at Edinburgh. American students received watered-down Monro and Cullen rather than original material based on the experiences of their own professors. In addition, the teachers apparently had little of the enthusiasm of their Edinburgh counterparts. Letters to the editor of the *National Gazette,* published in Philadelphia, indicate that this was clearly the case. In 1792, for instance, a writer noted that Dr. Benjamin Smith Barton was giving lectures on materia medica. Unfortunately, according to the author, the professor was dull and the teaching was presented in an "insipid dry & harsh manner." He concluded that any students who came to Philadelphia seeking a medical education would be sadly disappointed. They would feel like the proverbial Scotsman who had studied at Edinburgh, but who, after having paid the teacher, "left the university as ignorant as he came there." The writer predicted that Barton's students would exclaim about their professor: "The Devil take him; he is got more from me than I ever got from him."[37]

Less than a week after the first letter appeared in the *Gazette,* another one was published, this time signed by "Peter Plagiary." The letter began: "Odds Boddkins! Mr. Printer, why all this pother concerning the medical lectures of Late? Why not save the students of medicine the trouble of travelling three or four hundred miles?" The writer explained how to write a typical lecture presented at the American schools. First, it was necessary to "transcribe *verbatim*" from Sir William Temple's essay on health and long life. Then, the lecturer should read to his class from Cullen's works on fevers. "As the book is scarce, and as two thirds of your hearers will not be greatly distinguished for a retentive faculty, you will run little danger of being detected." The third bit of advice was to "never alter your opinion . . . it is always the sign of a weak mind; be inflexible, for an old error is better than a new truth."[38]

In addition to the problem of maintaining a high caliber of teaching in an area deficient in educated and experienced practitioners, public attitudes against dissection hindered the truly scientific study of medicine. In 1765, for example, when William Shippen was about to start his course of lectures, a rumor spread through Philadelphia that he had removed bodies from the church burying ground. Shippen responded in the *Pennsylvania Gazette,* dismissing the allegation of those "evil-minded persons" as "absolutely false." All the bodies that had been dissected in demonstrations for his students, he declared, either "had wilfully murdered themselves, or were publickly executed, except now and then one from the Potters Field, whose Death was owing to some particular Disease."[39] Thus, the "better class" of citizens had nothing to fear. The graves of their dearly departed relatives would not be touched.

In late 1787 or early 1788 Alexander Humphreys, the preceptor of Ephraim McDowell, had problems over a similar rumor. An Englishman visiting Staunton, Virginia, mysteriously disappeared. Later, while the citizenry was wondering about his whereabouts, a bag containing human remains was found in a cave. Suspicion naturally centered on Humphreys, who had a number of apprentices and who was known to be teaching anatomy. Humphreys' response was reminiscent of that of Shippen. He claimed that his students had dug up the body of a Negro, put it in a bag, and hid it in a cave. Local society had nothing to fear; it was only the body of a Negro![40]

From contemporary descriptions, however, it seems that the populace did have something to fear. Peter La Terriere, who had graduated from Harvard in 1789, described how Harvard students procured subjects. An old lady "both large and interestingly muscular" was buried in the graveyard of Christ Church. The beadle informed friends at the college, and he agreed to dig a shallow grave and leave a shovel near it. Thirty students descended on the cemetery at night and "carried off the prize in a large sack." According to La Terriere, there was a great deal of excitement when it was discovered that the grave had been disturbed, but Governor John Hancock, who was also president of the college's board of overseers, quashed the proceedings, and the excitement died down.[41] This episode was not reported in local newspapers, but it seems authentic, although perhaps somewhat exaggerated.

Harvard's search for cadavers was so intensive that, according to Edward Warren's *Life of John Collins Warren,* guards were posted in New England cemeteries to ward off the body snatchers. Warren described how bodies were dug up, starting in 1796, when he participated in such activities, and how bodies were snatched before burial by substituting logs for cadavers in the coffins. In cases of the latter, the students and professors had to be extremely careful; cemetery caretakers complained that it was embarrassing to have the log roll around in the coffin while being carried down the steps of the church or during the actual burial.[42]

That physicians did occasionally raid graveyards searching for subjects for dissection was not the only source of criticism. The medical profession, like its European counterpart, also came in for a great deal of criticism for providing inadequate medical treatment. At the time, treatment, which was far from effective, consisted of bloodletting and the administration of large doses of potentially dangerous drugs. It was popularly believed that physicians were almost as dangerous as the diseases they were called upon to combat. In 1755 William Douglass noted in his history of the American settlements that "it is better to let nature under a proper regimen take her course . . . than to trust the honesty and sagacity of the practitioner; our American practitioners," he exclaimed, "are so rash and officious" that the biblical admonition may be applied: "He that sinneth before his maker, let him fall into the hands of the physician."[43]

The popular suspicion of the medical profession, combined with the audacity of the colleges in their search for cadavers, led to violence in the famous New York doctors' riot in 1788. A group of medical students "ravaged" a cemetery for blacks, leading to a series of letters-to-the-editor by outraged citizens. Rather than denying the grave robbing, a medical student wrote a response to the letters appearing in the *Daily Advertiser.* He complained that "Humanio," who had written a letter condemning the editor (who had expressed sympathy for the "impassive bones of the dead"), was "either the most credulous of fools; or an infamous inventor of falsehoods." "For my own part," the student exclaimed, "I take thee to be the most stupid of asses." The student asked: "Whence is skill in surgery to be derived? And to whom would Humanio call for assistance, should he snap his leg, or burst a blood vessel?" He answered: "Run, run (he would say) to that barbarous man who has dissected most flesh, and anatomized most bone."[44]

As public opinion became more and more aroused at the indiscretions of the professors and the students, the situation fast got out of hand. The actual riot began when some young surgeons at the New York Hospital dangled a partially dissected limb from a window, calling to a young boy playing below that it was his mother's arm. The boy, whose mother had recently died, told his father. Upon investigation at the graveyard, the fellow discovered that his wife's grave had indeed been disturbed. He gathered his friends, who soon became a vicious mob. The result was four days of wanton destruction in a full-scale riot aimed at the medical profession and the college.

An excellent eyewitness account is found in the *Maryland Journal and Baltimore Advertiser.* It was in the form of a letter from New York, dated April 16, 1788. The letter began: "Our doctors by their imprudence and *indecency* in digging up, and *exposing* the *dead,* excited the rage of the populace." On Sunday, a mob gathered and "attacked the *Hospital*—dispersed the *Students* at *Physic*— destroyed all their preparations, etc." The mayor had to put the students into jail for their own protection. The following day, the mob gathered "in the fields" and paraded through the city, attacking the offices of leading physicians. The governor dispatched a company of militia, but the mob "broke their muskets and dispersed them." Then, according to the eyewitness who was a member of the militia, a larger body of soldiers and citizens gathered "at the burnt church" at six in the evening, led by the governor and General Malcom. The rioters let the soldiers go into the jail yard, but then "began a heavy fire upon us," as the account continued, "with *stones, bricks* and clubs, which so enraged our party, that we began a gentle fire upon them with muskets in return, which soon set them a running." The mob was not so easily deterred, however. They soon "returned to the

charge—and drove us fairly off the ground,—which they kept possession of till twelve o'clock at night, when they retired." At this
point, the doctors' riot of 1788 came to an end.[45]

The correspondent asserted in conclusion that "our doctors have
been very much to blame, and *magistrates* equally so, in permitting
them to act as they have done. The citizens, in general, appeared
unwilling to act on either side—They wished to see the physicians
suffer a little, and at the same time were opposed to the *mode of
redress.*"[46]

In the aftermath of the riot, a grand jury was impanelled to
investigate the charges that the physicians had engaged in grave
robbing. To indicate the state of public opinion on the matter and the
low esteem given to the medical profession, Chief Justice Morris'
charge to the jury began with the statement: "If this report is founded
in truth, which undoubtedly it is . . . ."[47] Until the medical profession improved its methods of treatment and acted in a more responsible manner, public opinion would look on the physicians as an
evil-minded group of men with no concern for the feelings of others.

Although the early medical schools had problems acquiring cadavers for dissection and demonstrations and although the colleges'
existence seemed precarious at times, such as during the doctors' riot
of 1788, the schools at Philadelphia, New York, and Boston were the
start of a great reform movement, a movement that was to be continued in the early nineteenth century with the establishment of
similar schools throughout the ever-expanding United States.

Notes

1. For a complete description of the establishment and operations of the
first medical college, see George W. Corner, *Two Centuries of Medicine: A
History of the School of Medicine, University of Pennsylvania* (Philadelphia,
1965). See also George W. Corner, "Beginnings of Medical Education in
Philadelphia, 1765-1776," *Journal of the American Medical Association* 194
(November 15, 1965): 719-721; Genevieve Miller, "Medical Schools in the
Colonies," *Ciba Symposia* 8 (January 1947): 522-532. For listings of faculty
changes, see Joseph Carson, *History of the Medical Department of the
University of Pennsylvania* (Philadelphia, 1869).

2. Whitfield J. Bell, Jr., *John Morgan: Continental Doctor* (Philadelphia, 1965), pp. 72-73. See also Whitfield J. Bell, Jr., "John Morgan," *Bulletin of the History of Medicine* 22 (September-October 1948): 543-561, and Peter D. Olch, "The Morgan-Shippen Controversy," *Review of Surgery* 22 (January-February 1965): 1-8.

3. Betsy Corner and C. C. Booth, *Chain of Friendship: Selected Letters of Dr. John Fothergill of London, 1735-1780* (Cambridge, Massachusetts, 1971), pp. 224-227. See also James E. Gibson, *Dr. Bodo Otto and the Medical Background of the American Revolution* (Springfield, Ill., 1937), p. 45.

4. Thomas Ruston to Job Ruston, Edinburgh, September 30, 1764, Ruston Papers, Library of Congress.

5. Ibid., London, February 4, 1767, April 11, 1767, Ruston Papers.

6. Nathan S. Goodman, *Benjamin Rush: Physician and Citizen* (Philadelphia, 1934), pp. 29-32.

7. *Pennsylvania Gazette,* November 11, 1762.

8. Bell, *John Morgan,* pp. 112-118; *Pennsylvania Gazette,* May 9, September 25, 1765.

9. John Morgan, *A Discourse upon the Institution of Medical Schools in America* (Philadelphia, 1765), p. 20.

10. Ibid., pp. 23-24.

11. Ibid., pp. 28-29, 36.

12. Ibid., p. 35.

13. *Pennsylvania Chronicle and Universal Advertiser,* July 27-August 3, 1767.

14. Ibid.

15. *Boston Chronicle,* July 4-11, 1768. For more details on the commencement, see *Pennsylvania Gazette,* June 30, 1768.

16. Bell, *John Morgan,* pp. 143-44. See also Elizabeth H. Thomson, "Thomas Bond, 1713-84," *Journal of Medical Education* 33 (1958): 614-624.

17. Bell, *John Morgan,* pp. 134-135.

18. For a complete description of the founding and operations of the King's College Medical School, see John Brett Langstaff, *Doctor Bard of Hyde Park* (New York, 1942); Byron Stookey, *A History of Colonial Medical Education in the Province of New York, with its Subsequent Development (1767-1830)* (Springfield, Illinois, 1962).

19. John Watts to General Robert Monckton, New York, May 16, 1764, cited in Langstaff, *Doctor Bard,* pp. 75-76.

20. *New-York Mercury,* September 7, 1767.

21. Byron Stookey, "America's Two Colonial Medical Schools," *Bulletin of the New York Academy of Medicine* 40 (April 1964): 279. The college held

held anatomy classes in 1765, revived by Clossy. See *New-York Mercury,* March 11, 1765.

22. *New-York Mercury,* November 9, 1767; Peter Middleton, *A Medical Discourse, or an Historical Inquiry into the Ancient and Present State of Medicine* (New York, 1769).

23. Stookey, "America's Two Colonial Medical Schools," 269-284.

24. Langstaff, *Doctor Bard,* pp. 102-103.

25. See *Boston Evening Post and General Advertiser,* September 13, 1783.

26. Thomas F. Harrington, *The Harvard Medical School* (New York and Chicago, 1904), I: 77-79.

27. Edward Warren, *Life of John Warren, M.D.* (Boston, 1874), pp. 245-251.

28. Harrington, *Harvard Medical School,* I: 84-85.

29. *Boston Evening Post and General Advertiser,* September 13, 1783.

30. Ibid. See also September 20, 1783, for a letter to the editor complaining about shortcomings in the Harvard plan for medical education.

31. Ibid., October 11, 1783.

32. *Continental Journal and Weekly Advertiser* (Boston), November 27, 1783.

33. *Massachusetts Spy* (Worcester), September 15, 1785.

34. Reginald Fitz, "The Surprising Career of Peter La Terriere, Bachelor in Medicine," *Annals of Medical History,* 3d ser. 3 (September 1941): 405-406.

35. Eugene F. Cordell, *Historical Sketch of the University of Maryland School of Medicine* (Baltimore, 1891), pp. 2-3; *Maryland Journal and Baltimore Advertiser* (extra), November 13, 1789.

36. *Maryland Journal and Baltimore Advertiser,* April 9, 13, 1790.

37. *National Gazette* (Philadelphia), October 20, 1792.

38. Ibid., October 24, 1792.

39. *Pennsylvania Gazette,* September 25, 1765.

40. Case cited in August Schachner, *Ephraim McDowell* (Philadelphia and London, 1921).

41. Quoted in Fitz, "Surprising Career of Peter La Terriere," 401.

42. Edward Warren, *Life of John Collins Warren* (Boston, 1860), I: 404ff.

43. William Douglass, *A Summary, Historical and Political, of the First Planting, Progressive Improvements, and Present State of the British Settlements in North-America* (London, 1755), quoted in John Blake, "Diseases and Medical Practice in Colonial America," *International Record of Medicine* 171 (June 1958): 359-60.

44. See *Daily Advertiser* (New York), February 23, 28, 29, March 1, 1788.

45. *Maryland Journal and Baltimore Advertiser,* April 25, 1788.

46. Ibid. See also the description and analysis in John Duffy, *A History of Public Health in New York City, 1625-1866* (New York, 1968), pp. 87-88.

47. *Daily Advertiser* (New York), April 17, 1788.

3

The Decline of American Medical Education

By 1813 seven medical colleges had been chartered and were in operation in the United States. The earliest schools, which remained from the late eighteenth century, had been branches of colleges of arts and sciences. The University of Pennsylvania, Harvard, King's College, and Dartmouth were all in this category. For the most part, these early colleges provided the best medical education possible outside of the European medical centers. Although in many cases the professors tended to be young and inexperienced graduates of European schools, they were the best available instructors. Moreover, the existence of such colleges made it possible to improve upon training by apprenticeship.

In the early years of the nineteenth century, four new schools were established. These were the College of Physicians and Surgeons in New York City, the University of Maryland, Yale University, and the College of Physicians and Surgeons of the Western District of New York. Of these, Yale was the only one with a collegiate connection. The others were established either by medical societies or by private practitioners.

The College of Physicians and Surgeons was a direct competitor of the medical department of Columbia College. King's College, which was established by Samuel Bard, suspended operations with the American Revolution, and it was finally abandoned when the faculty "scattered abroad."[1] In 1784 the state legislature created the regents of the University of the State of New York, who were to charter colleges and confer degrees on graduates of those colleges. The regents who were appointed did not establish a medical college until seven years later. In 1791 Dr. Nicholas Romayne asked the regents to consider his private "college" as the medical department of the university. Romayne, who evidently took the concept of preceptor seriously, had been lecturing on the various medical subjects, and in addition he had given clinical lectures at the Almshouse and at Bridewell. All the elements of a medical college existed in Romayne's private school. The members of the regents' committee who visited it were so impressed that they reported favorably on his petition.

"A movement in Columbia College," however, "defeated Dr. Romayne's plans."[2] In 1792 Columbia organized a medical faculty, which included Samuel Bard, John R. B. Rogers, and several other leading physicians. The college, which seems to have been established to thwart the plans of Dr. Romayne, was almost a total failure. Only thirty-five students graduated from its inception to 1811.

In 1806 the legislature passed a law establishing county medical societies, and at this point the stage was set for a competing college, which was sponsored by the Medical Society of the County of New York. Nicholas Romayne was president of that society, and his influence is clearly visible in the entire venture. On March 12, 1807, in spite of the opposition of Columbia College, the regents granted a charter to the College of Physicians and Surgeons of the University of the State of New York.[3]

The faculty included Romayne, Samuel Latham Mitchill, David Hosack, and Benjamin DeWitt. Soon the college was in full operation, attracting more students than had ever enrolled in a medical class in the city.[4] In 1814 the College of Physicians and Surgeons absorbed the medical department of Columbia College.[5] The resulting institution was to be filled with discord and dissension, which at times developed into open warfare between the various factions. The history of the college was one of rivalry, which often threatened to destroy it and establish competing schools.[6]

Indeed, Romayne's participation seemed to ensure that the college would not remain a quiet academic institution. Feuds and rivalries seemed to follow him wherever he went. He had spent time in prison for playing a role in Blount's 1797 conspiracy to raise a legion of militia and to both incite the Indians and aid the British in taking the Louisiana Territory from France and Spain. He has been called the "Stormy Petrel of American Medical Education"; his schools were characterized by rivalries that at times simmered below the surface but that periodically flashed into the open with pamphlet wars and with the secession of members of the faculty and the establishment of competing schools, like that at Rutgers College.[7]

In 1807, the year that the College of Physicians and Surgeons received its charter, medical education in the state of Maryland got its start when the College of Medicine of Maryland was established. It grew out of private lectures offered by two young physicians, John B. Davidge, a graduate of the University of Glasgow who had practiced in Birmingham, England, before returning to Maryland, and Nathaniel Potter, a product of the University of Pennsylvania and an ardent follower of Benjamin Rush. In 1807 they planned a full course of lectures with two more men, James Cocke, a graduate of the Philadelphia school who had also studied with Sir Astley Cooper at Guy's Hospital in London, and John Shaw, who had studied both at Philadelphia and Edinburgh.[8]

Davidge built a small anatomical theatre and managed to procure a cadaver, but the popular disapproval of dissection rose to plague the endeavor. A gang of boys gathered into a mob and destroyed the building. This proved not a disaster but rather a lesson for the physicians. It was obvious that they had to procure a charter, which would give them legal protection in the future. In December 1807 a charter was granted, placing the college in the hands of the state board of medical examiners, which operated much as a state medical society. The first class began immediately; there were only seven students, and lectures were given in the houses of the professors. It was a faltering start but a successful one. Soon the college was called the University of Maryland Medical School, and it would become a rival of the University of Pennsylvania.[9]

After the War of 1812, America's newly established medical colleges tended to be proprietary. They were chartered by a few physicians, often in a small rural village that had little or no clinical facilities. Traditionally historians have suggested that the proliferation of proprietary colleges resulted in a drastic reduction of standards, a reduction that destroyed the prestige of the medical profession, to say nothing of the effect on the citizens who were to become the "victims" of poorly trained physicians. The evidence indicates clearly, though, that the reduction of standards preceded the development of the proprietary school. For instance, in 1792 the University of Pennsylvania abolished the Bachelor of Medicine degree and substantially reduced the requirements for the Doctor of Medicine degree. No longer did the professors demand preliminary education in mathematics, the natural sciences, and Latin. Instead they required previous instruction in "Natural and Experimental Philosophy," which did not include mathematics and Latin and which was a giant step away from the traditional classical curriculum. No longer did it take seven years of practice after receiving the bachelor's degree to qualify for the doctorate. Interestingly, the M.D. degree required less work than previously had been required for the M.B. degree.[10]

The reduction of standards was necessary because of conditions in frontier America. Many potential students lived in rural areas, and attendance at medical school was time-consuming and expensive. As a result, most young men aspiring to become physicians either would not bother to attend college or they would attend only long enough to receive the bachelor's degree. They would practice medicine immediately upon completing their apprenticeships or after having received a bachelor's degree, and they would never aspire to the higher honors of the doctorate. With the elimination of the bachelor's degree, there would be a clearer distinction between trained and untrained practitioners. It would become worthwhile to attend college, receive a doctorate, and enter practice with prestige that could be acquired in a short period of time rather than the seven-year minimum required earlier for the doctorate.

Frederick Waite has analyzed the evolution of medical degrees in colonial America, and he provides some excellent statistics. The College of Philadelphia awarded twenty-nine bachelor's degrees in medicine from 1768 to 1774, and only five students returned to defend their theses and receive the doctorate. A similar situation existed at the University of Pennsylvania. It awarded sixty-seven bachelor's degrees from 1780 to 1791, and only six advanced M.D. degrees. At King's College, twelve students received the M.B. degree from 1768 to 1774, while only two students received the advanced M.D. degree. At Harvard, from 1783 to 1800, a total of twenty-nine students received the M.B. degree, and only one student returned for the advanced M.D. degree.[11]

In addition to the elimination of the bachelor's degree and its replacement by the doctorate, there was a reduction in the length of the medical course. At first, the term lasted from seven to nine months. When it became apparent that many students could not afford to live in the city and study for such a long period of time, the colleges began to reduce their courses to four and five months. This happened at Yale College. When it first opened in 1813, Yale offered a six-month course of medical lectures. Soon, because of competition with other schools, the time was reduced to five and then to four months. Students were being very selective; they flocked to those colleges that offered the M.D. degree in the shortest period of time.[12]

Events of the early and mid-nineteenth century were to compound the problem of decreasing standards of medical education. During this period, the relatively small number of medical schools multiplied; twenty-six new schools were established from 1810 to 1840, and forty-seven more were added from 1840 to 1877. By 1876 there were sixty-four medical colleges still in operation out of the eighty that had been established in the United States.[13]

These new schools were generally of the proprietary type established by a few local physicians, chartered by the state, and often operating without the facilities for proper medical training. Some of the proprietary schools received the wholehearted support of citizens of newly settled frontier towns. The college gave them a sense of pride; with a college present, they could consider their town a seat of knowledge, much like Boston, New York City, or Philadelphia. Daniel Boorstin, the social historian, has pointed out how local pride encouraged the establishment of western and southern colleges, colleges that local inhabitants considered equal to the best institutions of higher education on the eastern seaboard.[14] As long as the professors did not disturb the graves of former residents, they could count on the complete support of the community.

Most small-town colleges were developed by one or two leading physicians who decided for a number of reasons that it would be beneficial to establish a medical school. First, they could increase their incomes through student fees. They could also add to their practices by gaining a competitive advantage over other local physicians who could not advertise a college affiliation. Finally, being a professor in the medical school would increase the physician's sense of personal identity and prestige, no small matter in a time when the prestige of the profession was decreasing.[15]

Frederick Waite provides a fine description of the history of Castleton Medical College in Vermont, which was the first proprietary institution in New England.[16] Selah Gridley, a local physician, was the leader in the drive to establish the college. Although not a medical graduate himself, Gridley had a number of apprentices. The college would be a convenience for his students, enabling them to avoid the 150-mile trip to the College of Physicians and Surgeons of the Western District of New York, in Fairfield, Herkimer County. Yet, according to Waite, the stimulus for these small-town colleges was clearly financial. He describes how they scheduled their sessions to allow students to take one term elsewhere, transfer to Castleton, and receive the M.D. degree in eight months of study. This system could double the income of the professors, as the college would also have a second term in the same year.[17]

In addition to the pecuniary reasons for founding a college, it was burdensome for a country physician to have apprentices and private students; they interfered with a busy practice. If a number of preceptors could unite, each teaching a specialty, they could provide more efficient medical education for the students. At the same time, they would ensure that the money of their students would remain with them rather than ending up in the pockets of professors in Philadelphia or Boston. In addition, they would gain the prestige of being medical professors. In many cases, the quality of education was secondary to the benefits provided to the faculty. Thus, we find literally hundreds of complaints about the low level of medical training at the proprietary colleges.

Andrew Boardman described his experience with one of these

institutions, the Geneva Medical College in upstate New York. During demonstrations in the amphitheater, only those students in the front row could see what was happening. Those who *really* wanted to learn medicine had to enroll in a private class where they could observe demonstrations clearly. Boardman pointed out that the circular of the college mentioned that students would take a course of lectures in physiology and medical jurisprudence. After enrolling they would discover that it consisted of one insufficient lecture. The circular boasted of ample subjects for dissection, yet *"not a single subject* was provided." The circular said that students could attend clinical instruction at the Western Hospital. When the students arrived, they found the hospital on the second floor of a building labeled "Geneva Shoe Store," and it contained *"not one* medical patient, and *only one* surgical patient." Boardman, who served as house surgeon, stated that his daily rounds could be easily performed "by going from one side of the bed of a quiet old negress to the other."[18]

Because so many colleges were being established, it was difficult for most of them to turn a profit. There were too many colleges for the number of potential medical schools; instead of competing to provide the best training, they competed to provide the fastest, cheapest, and easiest education. The college that could make good on its claims to do all three could plan on having its benches filled to overflowing.

There are abundant records of violent cutthroat competition between the various colleges. For instance, the medical college at Willoughby, near Lake Erie, in northern Ohio, ran a battle with medical men and local citizens from Cleveland. In 1843 the entire faculty of the Willoughby school determined to move to Cleveland, obviously encouraged by the advantages of being in a major city where clinical resources would be more readily available. They were also impelled by the possibility of attracting more students, thus increasing their compensation.[19] The Cleveland Medical College was established by the resigning professors after they had gained an affiliation with Western Reserve College. Western Reserve would grant medical degrees to students recommended by J. P. Kirtland, John Delamater, David Long, and Erastus Cushing, the medical faculty.[20]

In November 1843 it was discovered that the officers of the Willoughby school were spreading rumors that Western Reserve could not legally grant medical degrees, an allegation that Dean J. L. Cassels of the Cleveland school denied.[21] The rumors continued to plague the new college. The students of the Cleveland Medical College held a mass meeting and adopted a series of resolutions expressing their anger at the fact that so many people were actively "engaged in carrying out their designs to mislead." The resolution declared that a majority of the physicians in the Western Reserve "regard Cleveland as the only place in northern Ohio fit—because of size, situation, and commercial importance—for a medical school" and that the professors "did right in severing connections with the 'Willoughby University of Lake Erie,' " "which was in Notorious and intimate union with the Ohio Rail Road Company."[22]

The following February, 1844, an editorial in the *Cleveland Herald* indicated that Willoughby had "erected a medical school with the expectation that with the Ohio railroad, the village would become very prosperous, but the one has failed and the other is about to follow."[23] Finally, in 1846 the Willoughby school was moved to Columbus, where it would have more clinical instruction, as well as the ability to attract more students.[24]

The story of the life of Daniel Drake includes a mass of material on rivalries both between colleges and within individual faculties. Early in his career, while at Transylvania, animosity developed between William H. Richardson, professor of obstetrics, and Benjamin W. Dudley, professor of anatomy and surgery. In 1818, as a result of mutual attacks and condemnations that violated the honor of each, the two professors agreed to fight a duel. Dudley wounded Richardson and then ministered to his adversary's wounds. Drake took up his pen in support of Richardson; in his *Second Appeal,* he bitterly questioned Dudley's integrity. He declared that "the ensigns of Paris foppery" had "nearly obscured the slender stock of intellect on which they were engrafted," and that "egotism, ignorance and sycophancy had formed within him an unholy alliance, and alternately guided the helm of his destinies."[25] Drake left Transylvania the following year to establish the Medical College of Ohio in Cincinnati. Considering Dudley's shooting ability, Lexington, Kentucky, was not a safe place for Drake to live.

In his inaugural address in 1820, Drake made a plea for improved standards of preliminary education of medical students and called for a general reform of medical education. He advocated lengthening the course to five months, and he emphasized the need for bedside teaching and hospital attendance. Due to Drake's influence, the Commercial Hospital and Lunatic Asylum was established in 1821 as a teaching hospital, staffed by the professors of the Medical College of Ohio.[26]

Then a bitter dispute developed, and Drake was dismissed by vote of the faculty, despite the fact that he was the founder of the school and that to a large extent the reputation of the school rested on his participation. In 1823 he returned to Transylvania, which was hardly the epitome of tranquillity. In 1830 and 1831 he was back in Ohio, trying to develop a new medical school affiliated with Miami University that would compete with the Medical College of Ohio. A court fight ensued over the charter, while the trustees of the existing college offered positions to Drake's entire faculty, including Drake, in order to prevent competition.[27]

Meanwhile dissension continued at Transylvania. Charles Caldwell was upset at his inability to procure sufficient anatomical material in Lexington, a problem that plagued other small-town institutions. In 1837 he sponsored a drive to transfer the college to Louisville. The trustees responded by dismissing Caldwell. Two other faculty members, John E. Cooke, professor of the theory and practice of medicine, and Lunsford P. Yandell, professor of chemistry, were so angry at the cavalier treatment accorded Caldwell that they joined him in the newly established Louisville Medical Institute. The Louisville school promised greater financial security than had the positions at Transylvania, along with improved clinical resources. Each professor's ticket (which would admit students to classes) cost fifteen dollars; if the college could attract 200 students, each professor would gross $3,000. In addition, a "chair assured all the private patients a professor could handle." Most of the faculty supplemented their incomes by taking private pupils and offering summer courses. In 1839 Daniel Drake was added to the Louisville faculty, and in 1840 Samuel D. Gross, the great anatomist, pathologist, and surgeon, joined him. At that point, the college had an exceptionally strong faculty.[28]

Perhaps the most interesting rivalry was the one between Benjamin Lincoln of the University of Vermont College of Medicine and Theodore Woodward of the Castleton Medical College. Lincoln was so appalled by the unethical actions of his competitor that he began to publicize the abuses his rival perpetrated. He documented the "crimes" committed by Woodward, who responded, leading to a long and bitter pamphlet war. Lincoln declared that Woodward had been guilty of publishing "false or extravagant circulars . . . to deceive students" and inventing "calumnious falsehoods against the officers of other schools and the telling of these falsehoods to Medical Students for the purpose of securing their attendance." He had dispatched "secret, confidential agents into the region round about to look up Pupils," and he authorized them to underbid competing schools, reduce requirements, and agree to examine students before completion of their three-year course of study.[29] Lincoln specifically accused Woodward of having enticed four Canadians to enroll at Castleton, and he documented how they were persuaded not to attend the University of Vermont.[30]

One of the most memorable episodes of intrafaculty rivalry occurred in 1856 and revolved around a faculty dispute over control of the Eclectic Medical Institute of Cincinnati. The dispute became so hot that it actually led to open and violent warfare between the two factions. At one point there were two armies of students and faculty members confronting each other with knives, pistols, bludgeons, and blunderbusses. The faction that held the building faced a siege by the opposing forces. According to reports, the tall and bewhiskered Professor Joseph Rodes Buchanan, a leading exponent of phrenology, urged his troops to the battle crying, "On on my lads." Finally the siege was broken when a six pound cannon was located and used to defend the building; the sight of the cannon dispersed the forces. The rest of the battle was fought in court.[31]

The intense rivalries between colleges, as well as the intense intrafaculty disputes, paved the way for the further deterioration of the quality of medical education. The problem began at the level of the preceptor. According to Dr. Daniel Holmes of Smithfield, Pennsylvania, "private practitioners" made a habit of receiving "uneducated and frequently unworthy young men into their office, for the sole purpose of benefitting themselves, by having their office drudgery done, books kept, accounts collected—or expecting by their means to gain friends, and thereby secure more patients." To keep their clientele, he said, some physicians even "give certificates of study to young men who have never entered their office at all, or grant certificates for a much longer time than they actually have studied."[32]

He told about a young man who had come into his office to inquire about the possibility of receiving a scholarship to medical school. The fellow had "read medicine" for four months without a preceptor, and a local physician had recommended that he attend a course of lectures in the winter and begin his practice in the spring. The physician had told him that "attending lectures was partially a humbug—more for the name than for the game—as one could learn nearly as much, and sometimes more, by reading and practice at home, and that it was useless to spend so much time to be admitted into the profession, for it would not pay."[33]

The evidence indicates that a great many medical students held those beliefs. For instance Charles William Cary, who graduated from the Jefferson Medical College in 1851, described in his diary why he selected that school: he considered the professors "as abler men, being younger"; the session was "a month shorter than that of the old school"; and he received a better offer from Jefferson. As "in consequence of having attended two courses of lectures elsewhere," he said, "I got into the 'Jeff' for half the amount of fees that I could have entered the other school for." Finally, his roommate decided to enroll, "and it was much more pleasant for both to belong to the same."[34] There was no comparison between Jefferson and its competitors, the University of Pennsylvania and the University of Virginia.

In an 1847 pamphlet, Daniel Drake described the various types of medical students. Among them were those who wanted only practical knowledge, as they intended to practice after the first course of lectures. Then there were those who were studying medicine "without possessing powers of mind adequate to that extended and difficult understanding." Finally there were those whose social interests would substitute "a love of sex for the love of science" and those whose morals were "dissipated," as well as a few "bullies and desperadoes."[35] Such was the result when the colleges competed desperately for students without paying attention to the backgrounds, character, or education of their applicants.

Drake offered a number of suggestions to the students. Foremost among them was to "forego the pleasures and amusements of the city." "The eye that is dancing with pleasure," he exclaimed, "or dull from its excess, sees but imperfectly the aspects of disease in the clinical wards." Students, he said, should "seek for recreation, not debauchery."[36] When students from rural backgrounds left the influence of their parents, however, the pursuit of knowledge was often cast into the background by the excitements, amusements, and entertainments of the city.

Indeed, the immoralities of the city provided ammunition for the advocates of country medical colleges. T. Romeyn Beck, for instance, wrote that city schools encouraged students to "indulge in vicious dissipation," while rural schools, being secluded, were "calculated to direct the mind to study."[37]

An example of immoralities at a city school can be seen in the early history of the University of Maryland at Baltimore. In December 1828 Nathaniel Potter became curious when he noticed several students entering the janitor's apartment. When he investigated, he was shocked to find several students "regaling themselves with spirits and cards." It seems that the janitor was adding to his income by selling whiskey to the students and letting them drink in the safety of his apartment. He apparently had a steady business.[38]

Rural schools were not exempt from such activities, however. At the University of Michigan at Ann Arbor, "many of the more adventurous students" frequented a local house of prostitution. Everyone seemed to be contented until disaster finally struck. One student fell in love with "an inmate" and while intoxicated promised to marry her. When he regained his senses, he decided to kill himself rather than bring such disgrace to his family. His death resulted in a mass meeting of students and a decision to run "old Mother Raphelgie" out of town. The students armed themselves with pistols and clubs and surrounded the house. The madam refused to leave town, declaring, "He that is without sin among you, let him first cast a stone at her." At that open invitation, a brick went crashing through a window. There was a "fusillade of shots" from the house in reply. The students dispersed and rallied for a charge; they rushed at the building, firing their pistols. The *Detroit Evening News* reported the incident as a "murderous assault by a mob of medical students upon a houseful of women." This episode was indicative of the rough type of student attracted to the medical profession in the nineteenth century.[39]

The colleges paid little attention to the character of their students and even less to their preliminary education. The major characteristic of the American college was a "total neglect of all examinations into the previous education and capacity of the student."[40] Even those students who were willing and able to devote themselves to the study of medicine had to face an environment that was not conducive to learning. They might be surrounded by men who were inadequately prepared or who were not capable of absorbing the material; they most likely were attending a college that did not have all of the needed apparatus and facilities. A fellow who attended Harvard during the 1825-1826 session described what had to be a most depressing environment. On a visit to the Massachusetts General Hospital for an observation of John C. Warren's operation for harelip, seventeen assistants blocked the view. "We could only discover the steps of the operation," the observer declared, "by the cries of the patient. The first incision was announced by an outcry, and the succeeding steps were traced by cries and now and then a *kick* of the patient by the operator."[41]

In another example of the problems facing the medical student of the day, Thomas S. Kirkbride, who was later to become an early psychiatrist and asylum superintendent, seemed to show little interest in the lectures he attended at the University of Pennsylvania Medical School from 1828 to 1831. According to his biographer, "He put down no notes; he recorded some of the stories told by the professors and jotted down a few lines of the jokes which enlivened their discourses." He took extensive notes only in surgery, and his notebooks included only two meager pages of notes on the physiology of the nervous system. Moreover, his thesis was based on notes he had made while working with his preceptor.[42] It seems that a great deal of the education of the nineteenth-century physician came while he was an apprentice or after his formal training had been completed.

W. K. Bowling, editor of the *Nashville Journal of Medicine and Surgery,* could easily recall his first session as a student in the late 1820s at the Medical College of Ohio. The college, Daniel Drake's institution, was considered one of the better schools in the country and certainly one of the two best in the West. Bowling's description was in the form of questions and answers. The first question was, "How many operations on live folks did you see the first course?" The answer was, "None." "Was there a hospital accessible to the students?" "Yes." "How often did you visit it?" "Twice." "What did you see the first time?" "A furious madman chained to a ring in the middle of his cell." "What did you see the second time?" "A man with the dropsy." "Was he benefitted by the treatment?" "He died." "What did you see the second course?" "Two operations on the eye. One was on a man, the other on a decapitated sheep."[43] With that amount of clinical work, he and his classmates were graduated, and they scattered to practice throughout the West.

The quality of education at the regular medical colleges was so bad that some established summer schools, which provided more personal contact with the professors than was possible in a large amphitheater filled with one hundred or more students. The summer classes were not required, and in some cases they attracted as many as one-third of the students. As early as 1827 Harvard's professors had developed private schools, and in 1838 they were formalized with the establishment of what became known as the Tremont Street Medical School, with Jacob Bigelow, Oliver Wendell Holmes, D. H. Storer, and Edward Reynolds on the faculty. It was not chartered by the state, but it provided private instruction and demonstrations in an atmosphere more conducive to teaching and learning.[44]

Unfortunately, the summer schools did not attract those students who could have profited most from special instruction. Only those who were affluent enough to attend (rather than work to finance their studies) could possibly enroll. And of those affluent ones, only those who seriously wanted to become professional physicians were willing to devote a summer of study; the others were happy to begin their practice and profit from their studies, in spite of obvious shortcomings. Looking at the summer schools from this perspective, it seems that the object was to add to the income of the professors as well as to benefit those students who could afford and who wanted better medical training than they received at the colleges.[45]

If one considers the accomplishments of the members of the various faculties, it would seem that they were well able to provide their students with a fine medical education. In 1825 the faculties included the top men in the American medical profession. Philadelphia had Philip Syng Physick, John Redman Coxe, and Nathaniel Chapman; New York City had David Hosack, Samuel Latham Mitchill, Valentine Mott, and John Wakefield Francis; Boston (Harvard) had John C. Warren, Walter Channing, James Bigelow, and James Jackson; Yale had Nathan Smith and Benjamin Silliman; Transylvania had Daniel Drake; and so on down the list.[46]

Yet scientific eminence and accomplishment can bear little relationship to teaching ability. The descriptions of the teachers in the classrooms are often quite revealing. In his two-volume autobiography, Samuel D. Gross described the medical lecturers of his time. Charles Meigs, professor of midwifery at the Jefferson Medical College, was "rarely, if ever, systematic." George McClellan, the founder of that school, was "brilliant, always interesting and instructive," but "superficial and scattering, apparently without any definite aim, forethought, or preparation." Daniel Drake was "a great lecturer," but "first course students . . . could never follow or understand him, because he always overshot his mark." According to Gross, some lecturers "are learned dunces," men who think they must give an opinion on everything that anybody ever wrote on a subject or who emphasize their own interests, however irrelevant to their subject. Dr. Short of the University of Louisville read his lectures and never looked up at his class. Charles Caldwell was a "model of a lecturer, walking to and fro upon the rostrum like a caged lion," but he was "a miserable teacher" and Gross doubted that he "ever made a physiologist of any of his pupils." William Dewees was one of the most authoritative and experienced teachers of obstetrics and gynecology, having delivered upwards of ten thousand women, but according to Gross his lectures were "unrefined . . . abounding in coarse anecdotes and sayings." He always lectured in the afternoons, "under the influence of vinous potations." Robley Dunglison "was always brimful of his subject," but "he was monotonous." John E. Cooke, "one of the dullest and most arid lecturers that could possibly be imagined," was nevertheless "a successful teacher." But there was an exception: Gross described Granville Sharp Pattison as "one of the most interesting lecturers of his day."[47]

Pattison's biography demonstrates that morality and "character" had little relationship to success as a medical educator. He arrived in America in 1819, and he inquired about joining the faculty of the University of Pennsylvania. Nathaniel Chapman discovered that he had left Scotland under embarrassing circumstances—in the aftermath of a divorce trial of a colleague who argued that Pattison had had improper relations with his wife. When Pattison learned that Chapman was spreading the story of the divorce scandal, he was outraged. He went to Philadelphia, publicly called Chapman a liar, a coward, and a scoundrel, and was arrested and held in custody for a short time. In 1820 Pattison challenged Chapman to a duel, which was refused. Later, Pattison fought a duel with General Thomas Cadwalader, Chapman's brother-in-law, who was severely wounded in the encounter. In addition to being plagued by his alleged escapades in Scotland, Pattison's health was reportedly so damaged by "his revels" in America that he was forced to dose himself with mercury, the traditional cure for syphilis.[48]

Obviously some of the instructors were fit for the task, being sufficiently knowledgeable and able to impart their knowledge to the students, as well as being examples of the higher morality expected of a follower of Hippocrates. On the other hand, some were unable to teach, regardless of their preeminence in medical science. The result, for the student, must have been disastrous, especially if we consider that many students came poorly prepared to benefit from an intensive four-, five-, or six-month course of medical lectures. Daniel Drake constantly complained that although the course was so short, "numerous students go home, before the expiration of the session." He figured that about one of every four students returned home without waiting for the course to come to an end. This could indicate that for these young men, the course was so difficult that it seemed ridiculous to remain, especially when one could practice without a degree.[49]

Medical science clearly attracted a lower class of student than did any other of the professions. A low percentage of medical students were graduates of colleges of arts and sciences. In 1850-1851, 80 percent of the theological students and 65 percent of law students, but only 26 percent of medical students held bachelor's degrees.[50]

Records of the early medical licensing boards attest to the inadequate preparation given to many of the medical students. On

November 13, 1849, Othniel H. Taylor, the vice-president of the Medical Society of New Jersey, reported that a great many students customarily failed the board examinations. In the process they often demonstrated none of the knowledge that would be expected of students of medical science. Taylor gave examples from his experiences in New Jersey. When a student was asked what an expectorant was, he responded, "I can't exactly tell." When asked if he would prescribe expectorants in his practice, the same young man replied, "Yes, Sir, by all means." Another student, who came to the examination with the "strongest letters of recommendation from the highly distinguished professors of his school," demonstrated quite "a degree of ignorance" under examination.[51]

In an issue of the *Western Journal of Medicine and Surgery* in 1840 it was reported that according to the United States Surgeon General, only five of twenty-two applicants for appointment as assistant surgeons in the army medical department were found to be qualified. All of the applicants were graduates of American medical schools. Daniel Drake editorialized that the problem was not simply the proliferation of the schools but the short sessions and the low compensation of physicians, which attracted a lower class than previously had been the case.[52]

It is quite difficult to generalize about the quality of education in America's medical schools. For some students, the schools provided an excellent conclusion to a firm foundation laid by the diligent preceptor. Other students, however, were mentally unprepared to benefit from medical lectures or they were morally unfit to be physicians. In comparison with the medical education of the past, it is clear that whatever their inadequacies, the schools provided at least the possibility of advanced medical training for those students who were willing to spend the time and energy acquiring it. This is the argument presented by Asa Lord, an Ohio physician, in an article in the *Ohio Medical and Surgical Journal.* Lord, writing in 1851, noted that in the recent past, especially in the frontier areas, "we were without such schools." The student had to study in the office of a practitioner and had to be content "with the small library it contained, and with such instruction as the business of his preceptor would permit him to communicate." Also, the difficulty of traveling to New York or Philadelphia forced a great many young men either to abandon the dream of being physicians or practice without adequate schooling. According to Lord, the medical colleges were a godsend to the outlying areas, enabling local students to get formal training and providing the citizenry with better practitioners.[53] Yet it was obvious to virtually every observer that the quality of medicine was decreasing as the fierce competition between the colleges increased.

Notes

1. Edward Delafield, "Sketch of the History of the College of Physicians and Surgeons of the University of the State of New York," extracted in *New York Journal of Medicine,* 3d ser. 2 (March 1857): 165.

2. Ibid., 165-166.

3. Ibid., 166-167. Rivalry between the colleges was rampant during this period. For evidence see John W. Francis, Report to the College of Physicians and Surgeons, May 5, 1815, John D. Jaques to Samuel L. Mitchill, Albany, February 3, 1820, and Lyman Spalding to John D. Jaques, New York, February 18, 1820, Special Manuscript Collections, College of Physicians and Surgeons, Columbia University.

4. See *New York Journal of Medicine,* 3d ser. 2 (March 1857): 167-168.

5. For details of the struggle that developed between Hosack and Romayne, see Joseph Kett, *The Formation of the American Medical Profession* (New Haven and London: Yale University Press, 1968), p. 38.

6. James McNaughton, "Address Delivered before the Medical Society of the State of New York, February 8th, 1837," abstract and review in *American Journal of the Medical Sciences* 20 (August 1837): 469-475.

7. Fred B. Rogers, "Nicholas Romayne, 1756-1817: Stormy Petrel of American Medical Education," *Journal of Medical Education* 35 (March 1960): 258-263. See also David Cowen, *Medical Education: The Queen's-Rutgers Experience, 1792-1830* (New Brunswick, New Jersey, 1966); Herman G. Weiskotten, "Nicholas Romayne: Pioneer in Medical Education in the United States," *New York State Journal of Medicine* 66 (August 15, 1966): 2158-2177.

8. Eugene F. Cordell, "Our Alma Mater in 1807," *Maryland Medical Journal* 7 (October 1, 1880): 251-255; and Eugene F. Cordell, *Historical Sketch of the University of Maryland School of Medicine* (Baltimore, 1891).

9. Ibid.

10. See, for instance, the analysis in N. S. Davis, *History of Medical*

Education and Medical Institutions in the United States of America (1851), pp. 50-55.

11. Frederick Waite, "Medical Degrees Conferred in the American Colonies and in the United States in the Eighteenth Century," *Annals of Medical History,* n.s. 9 (July 1937): 315-320.

12. See Whitfield Bell, Jr., "The Medical Institution of Yale College, 1810-1885," *Yale Journal of Biology and Medicine* 33 (December 1960): 172. See also Davis, *Contributions,* p. 43.

13. Davis, *Contributions,* p. 41.

14. Daniel J. Boorstin, *The Americans: The National Experience* (New York: Vintage Books, 1965), pp. 152-161.

15. Frederick Waite, "Birth of the First Independent Proprietary Medical School in New England, at Castleton, Vermont, in 1818," *Annals of Medical History,* n.s. 7 (May 1935): 242-252.

16. Ibid.

17. Frederick Waite, *The First Medical College in Vermont: Castleton, 1818-1862* (Montpelier, Vermont, 1949), pp. 83-84.

18. Andrew Boardman, *Essay on the Means of Improving Medical Education and Elevating Medical Character* (Philadelphia, 1840), pp. 5-7. For the early history of the Geneva school, see Betsy C. Corner, "Early Medical Education in Western New York, Geneva and Rochester Areas, 1827-1872," *New York State Journal of Medicine* 55 (November 1, 1955): 3156-3164.

19. *Cleveland Herald,* May 23, 1843.

20. Ibid., August 28, 1843.

21. Ibid., November 11, 1843.

22. Ibid., November 14, 1843.

23. Ibid., February 19, 1844.

24. Ibid., August 18, 1846.

25. Emmett Field Horine, *Daniel Drake* (Philadelphia, 1961), pp. 124-131.

26. Ibid., pp. 167-1 |0.

27. Ibid., pp. 255-256.

28. Hampden C. Lawson, "The Early Medical Schools of Kentucky," *Bulletin of the History of Medicine* 24 (March-April 1950): 170; Emmett Field Horine, *Biographical Sketch and Guide to the Writings of Charles Caldwell, M.D.* (Brooks, Kentucky, 1960), 11-12.

29. Benjamin Lincoln, *Hints on the Present State of Medical Education and the Influence of Medical Schools of New England* (Burlington, Vermont, 1833), p. 17; Benjamin Lincoln, *An Exposition of Certain Abuses Practiced by Some of the Medical Schools of New England and Particularly*

of the Agent-Sending System as Practiced by Theodore Woodward(Burlington, Vermont, 1833).

30. William A. R. Chapin, *History of the University of Vermont College of Medicine* (Burlington, Vermont, 1951), pp. 24-25. See also Benjamin Lincoln Papers, Countway Library, Harvard Medical School.

31. See Harvey W. Felter, *History of the Eclectic Medical Institute* (Cincinnati, 1902), pp. 41-42.

32. Daniel Holmes, "An Essay on Medical Education," *Transactions of the Medical Association of Southern Central New York*(Auburn, New York, 1854), p. 39. See also J. Berrien Lindsley, *On Medical Colleges*(Nashville, 1858), pp. 25-26, and Daniel Drake, *Practical Essays on Medical Education and the Medical Profession in the United States* (Cincinnati, 1832) for evidence of the deficiencies in the apprenticeship system.

33. Holmes, "An Essay on Medical Education," 41. A computer study indicates that of the physicians who practiced in six New England counties from 1790 to 1840, 70 percent had never attended medical lectures and only 25 percent were medical college graduates. See Barnes Riznik, "Medicine in New England, 1790-1840" (typescript, Sturbridge, Mass., 1963).

34. Diary of Charles William Cary, Feamster Family Papers, Library of Congress. More on the character of students can be seen in John D. Godman, *Monition to the Students of Medicine*(Philadelphia, 1825), and Thomas D. Mitchell, *The Professor and the Pupil* (Philadelphia, 1862).

35. Daniel Drake, *Strictures on Some of the Defects and Infirmities of Intellectual and Moral Character, in Students of Medicine* (Louisville, 1847), p. 9. S.P. Crawford, "Medical Education," *Nashville Journal of Medicine and Surgery* 12 (February 1857): 101-105, states that an illiterate physician "is no uncommon thing."

36. Daniel Drake, *An Introductory Lecture, on the Means of Promoting the Intellectual Improvement of the Students and Physicians, of the Valley of the Mississippi. Delivered in the Medical Institute of Louisville, November 4, 1844* (Louisville, 1844), pp. 4-5.

37. T. Romeyn Beck, *On the Utility of Country Medical Institutions* (Albany, 1825), pp. 18-19.

38. Cordell, *Historical Sketch,* pp. 81-82.

39. This episode took place in 1878. See James D. Wood, *An Old Doctor of the New School* (Caldwell, Idaho, 1942), pp. 133-135; Martin Kaufman, *Homeopathy in America* (Baltimore, 1971), p. 107.

40. Reynall Coates, *Oration on the Defects in the Present System of Medical Instruction in the United States* (Philadelphia, 1835), pp. 11-12.

41. Quoted in Anna C. Holt, "A Medical Student in Boston, 1825-26," *Harvard Library Bulletin* 6 (1952): 360.

42. Earl D. Bond, *Dr. Kirkbride and His Mental Hospital*(Philadelphia, 1947), pp. 22-23.

43. *Nashville Journal of Medicine & Surgery*, n.s. 4 (June 1869): 598-615.

44. Thomas F. Harrington, *The Harvard Medical School* (New York and Chicago, 1905), II: 495-500, III: 1004. See also Claire G. Fox, "Dr. Heber Chase: *The Medical Student's Guide,*" *Bulletin of the History of Medicine* 42 (September-October 1968): 462-469, which describes the private courses in Philadelphia.

45. In 1835 Yale instituted summer courses that were not required, attracting about one-third of the students. See Whitfield Bell, Jr., "The Medical Institution of Yale College, 1810-1885," *Yale Journal of Biology & Medicine* 33 (December 1960): 176.

46. See Thomas Sewall, *Lecture, Delivered at the Opening of the Medical Department of the Columbian College in the District of Columbia, March 30, 1825* (Washington, D.C., 1825), p. 68.

47. *Autobiography of Samuel D. Gross* (Philadelphia, 1887), I: 163ff.

48. Cordell, *Historical Sketch,* pp. 50-53.

49. *Western Journal of Medicine & Surgery* 7 (January 1843); 71.

50. Bell, "The Medical Institution of Yale College," 174.

51. Othniel H. Taylor, *Medical Reform and the Present System of Medical Instruction* (Camden, 1850); Othniel H. Taylor, in *Transactions, Medical Society of New Jersey, 1766-1858* (Newark, 1875), 482-483.

52. *Western Journal of Medicine and Surgery* 1 (May 31, 1840): 384-386.

53. Asa D. Lord, "Medical Education," *Ohio Medical and Surgical Journal* 4 (November 1851): 112-116.

4

The Heroic Age and the Growth of the Irregulars

The period from the 1790s to about 1850 has been designated by historians as the "age of heroic medicine." During those years summoning a physician almost certainly meant undergoing treatment that in an earlier or later time might be characterized as torture. Bleeding, blistering, cupping, purging, and sweating were the major techniques the medical profession used. In the 1760s and 1770s, except in cases of pleurisy and rheumatism, there was little bloodletting. By 1810 virtually every disease called for massive bloodletting, often until the patient lapsed into unconsciousness.[1]

Benjamin Rush provided much of the theoretical basis for the great increase in venesection. Although he had studied under William Cullen at Edinburgh, Rush came to reject Cullen's system of medical practice. Cullen had observed that there were three stages in fever: debility, chill, and heat. Correlating these with changes in the small blood vessels, he worked out treatments based on the stage and type of fever. Physicians tried to eliminate "spasm" from the extreme arteries through what was known as the "antiphlogistic regimen," a combination of rest, careful attention to diet, applications of cold substances, and purging and bloodletting to reduce the quantity of fluids.[2]

According to Rush's analysis, fever resulted from "irregular action or convulsion" of the blood vessels. Because there was only one cause of disease, there could be only one cure—bloodletting. Treatment, then, should be either depletion through bloodletting or stimulation through medication. The Philadelphia physician was so enthusiastic about venesection that he even advocated it to the extent of removing four-fifths of the patient's blood.[3]

Rush was on the faculty of the University of Pennsylvania when Philadelphia was the medical capital of the young nation. What was thought and taught at Philadelphia had a great impact upon American practice. This is especially true when one considers the fact that professors at the other colleges often were graduates of the University of Pennsylvania where they learned their medicine from Rush. Rush was a great influence; his students spread through the country advocating massive bloodletting and teaching the efficacy of venesection to their apprentices and to students at other medical schools.[4]

Any student attending Rush's lectures had to be impressed with his zeal in advocating the use of the lancet. He began the course in 1798 by insisting that his own system was far superior to that of William Cullen. He made an analogy comparing disease to a house containing one hundred rooms. According to Cullen, each room had a different lock and the physician had to have "an equal number of different Keys to open them." Rush proudly asserted: "I am capable of entering every apartment of my House with the assistance of a single Key." That key was bloodletting. Every lecture extolled the importance of the lancet in treating disease. Rush tried to convince his students that venesection was easy and safe. Bleeding, he said, "but once or twice . . . is like untying a Tyger & not destroying him afterwards." "'Tis a very hard Matter," he claimed, "to bleed a Patient to Death." Rush even defended himself against critics who ridiculed him for bleeding his patients "till they were as pale as Jersey Veal." He exclaimed: "I would sooner die with my Lancet in my hand than give it up while I had Breath to maintain it or a hand to use it." The remainder of the course consisted of descriptions of various diseases, along with the recommended treatment. In every case, the treatment consisted of bloodletting, even to the extent of one hundred to two hundred ounces.[5]

By 1810 the medical profession had adopted bloodletting as well as a drastic purgative known as "Rush's Thunderbolt," a combination of jalap (a powder derived from a plant root) and calomel (mercurous chloride). An analysis of contemporary textbooks attests to the widespread use of the practices Rush advocated.[6] As late as the 1878 edition of John B. Biddle's *Materia Medica for the Use of Students,* heroic medicine was still highly recommended. Biddle advised bloodletting by venesection or phlebotomy to moderate vascular excitement, reduce inflammation, relieve congestion, allay spasm and pain, relax the muscular system, and arrest hemorrhage. Biddle did include a warning that bloodletting should not be used indiscriminately and that it should "not be unduly repeated." Then he described the benefit of leeching in infants and bloodletting by cupping. He described various emetics used to induce vomiting, cathartics used to purge from the bowels, and the drastic cathartics, such as jalap and calomel.[7] In fairness to Rush and his colleagues, knowledge of pathology was defective, and medical teachers could offer their students only what they knew or thought they knew.

Private correspondence as well as physicians' records demonstrate both the use and the abuse of heroic medicine. In 1820 when Sarah Granger Monteith became ill, her husband, the Reverend John Monteith of Detroit, noted in his diary the complete details of her treatment. "My dear wife in critical health. Dr. Hanchett gives physic." Four days later, on September 19, she was "Taking Calomel." On September 21 there was a change in the prescribed treatment. "Dr. Wright applies some plasters, continuing calomel," and he bathed her feet in warm water. On the following day the reverend wrote that his wife had started to salivate, which was an early sign of mercury poisoning from an overdose of calomel. Over the next few days, Mrs. Monteith took a dose of sulphur and used magnesia and "calomel cathartick." On October 2, Dr. Wright called in a Doctor Case for consultation, and Case prescribed some pills to keep the bowels open, tea of valerian and castor oil as gentle stimulants, and warm drinks through the night. It seems that by October 4 Wright had given up on the moderate treatment, and he returned to apply blisters to the head and elsewhere. The next day Monteith sadly wrote that his wife had been "given up by all three doctors." Then he noted: "Blisters have drawn well, especially those on head. Her hair is shaved." Finally—and perhaps mercifully—she died on October 9.[8]

In 1827 Dr. William Prescott of Concord, New Hampshire, asked some of his colleagues what they prescribed for acute enteritis. The responses indicated that massive bloodletting was almost universally recommended. Indeed, the one physician who did not advocate venesection seemed apologetic for the fact that he did "not bleed so freely as many do in this disease, or [as] indiscriminately."[9]

Testimony from patients indicates that heroic medicine was rampant in the United States prior to the Civil War. In 1829, for instance, John P. Sheldon, of Detroit, suffered with a severe chest cold. He stayed with Dr. William Brown. In his private correspondence he described the treatment. "I began with a smart dose of Calomel and Jalap, which helped me very much." Then he had a relapse, which he attributed to the fact that the doctor told him to "eat hearty food" and gave him a "couple of pills of opium" to "allay" a cough. Then, perhaps beneficially, he was forced to provide much of his own treatment, as "the Doctor has taken it into his head to drink too much brandy, and is in one of his squalls."[10]

In 1832 Charles M. Bull described in a letter to his father how he was treated by his physician. "I was in the first place bled 3 times & Physicked almost to deth. I tole the Doct. that my constitution was weak. If I could have had the Doct. Merriman Jr. in the first place," he claimed, "I should have got along better, but he was taken down sick the same day that I was." Then, in the midst of the great cholera epidemic of 1832, Bull explained that "the Doctors have got an idea into their heads that they must give calomel for evry complaint." He exclaimed: "They have fed me so much on it since I have been hir that I have lost all of my hair from my head and a good share of my teeth."[11]

Dr. John E. Cooke, who taught at Transylvania University in Kentucky, wrote that Benjamin Rush had been "vilified" in his day for giving ten grains of purgative jalap, yet by 1833 "thousands of physicians administer up to 100 grains." Cooke was one of the strongest advocates of the heroic treatment. He is reported to have said: "If calomel did not salivate, and opium did not constipate, there is no telling what we could do in the practice of physic." In one case he administered thirteen tablespoons of calomel in three days in an attempt to alleviate an attack of cholera. The patient died. In his last illness Cooke purged himself thoroughly with calomel and bled himself copiously, all to no avail.[12]

In 1840 Emily Mason wrote to tell her sister that she had been "suffering with a terrible pain" in her face, "The result of cold." "Today," she said, "I am threatened with leeching—Don't you envy me having those sweet little worms in my mouth?"[13] The Reverend Theodore Clapp of New Orleans wrote that in epidemics he had personally witnessed a physician, on "his first visit to a patient, who had been ill but four hours, take from him, by the lancet, fifty ounces of blood at one time." The fellow had fainted, but even that did not protect him from his physician. When he revived, the doctor "then ordered him to swallow, at once, three hundred grains of calomel and gamboge [a resin derived from certain trees, used as a cathartic]."[14]

Interestingly, it seems that observers in every part of the nation attributed the failures of heroic medicine to physicians of other sections than their own. In 1833 a reviewer in the *Western Journal of Medical and Physical Sciences* stated: "The practice of our brethren of the lower Mississippi, is well known to be characterized by great boldness and energy. The lancet and calomel, particularly the last, constitute their anchor of hope, in the endemic fevers of that region."[15] Then, after Dr. John P. Harrison of Cincinnati read a paper before the Hamilton County Medical Club in 1845, a commentator said that Harrison "recommended herculian doses of Calomel & opium. . . . None but a Kentuckyan would give or take such doses." Yet one can assume that Harrison's Ohio patients followed their good doctor's advice, even if it meant undergoing the entire heroic regimen.[16]

There was some debate about the efficacy of the heroic treatment, but according to John Duffy, the historian of medicine in Louisiana, while the controversy raged, the average physician continued to bleed, blister, purge, and administer calomel and opium.[17] Heroic medicine was clearly part of the American scene, and it seemed to be "here to stay." It was even the subject of a humorous song by Jesse Hutchinson, one of America's leading songwriters.[18] "A Dose of

Calomel" demonstrates the public attitude toward the physicians of
the day and their heroic treatments:

> Physicians of the highest rank,
> To pay their fees would need a bank,
> Combine all wisdom, art and skill,
> Science and sense in—*Calomel.*
>
> The man grows worse quite fast indeed!
> Go, call the doctor, ride with speed;—
> The doctor comes, like post with mail,
> Doubling his dose of—*Calomel.*
>
> The man in death begins to groan,
> The fatal job for him is done!
> He dies alas! and sad to tell—
> A sacrifice to—*Calomel!*

An overdose of calomel, however, was hardly comical. Heroic
medicine undoubtedly contributed to the high mortality rate of the
day. Many of those who had already been weakened by illness died
during the heroic treatments. In addition, it can be assumed that
harsh therapeutics prolonged the suffering of many people who
would have improved had nature been allowed to take its course. An
example of this is found in the *Detroit Free Press* of December 23,
1859. An announcement stated that a Police Justice would not be
able to hold sessions of his court during the week, as he was suffering
from "the excessive use of calomel."[19]

The abuse of heroic practice, aside from its unfortunate effect on
public health, convinced Americans that it was safer to treat oneself
than to be attended by a physician. As one historian stated: "Not
every sick man felt like being a hero."[20] When people fell sick, they
sought alternate forms of treatment. They may have devoted more
time than usual to attempts at self-medication. Then, the inexpensive
newspapers of the Jacksonian period enabled nostrum venders to
advertise the benefits of their cure-alls, and they did so in terms of
the "gory symptoms, the glorious cures, the glowing testimonials" of

those who had undergone the cure, of course, emphasizing mild medication rather than the heroic practices of the orthodox profession.[21] A committee of the New Hampshire Medical Society reported in 1856 that "so strong an antagonistic feeling" between physicians and the public existed that the people "regard their reliance upon nostrums and quack administration of medicine more valuable than any dependence upon a learned profession."[22]

The widespread suspicion of the medical profession was compounded when many Americans had adverse experiences with itinerent practitioners who took advantage of the shortcomings of the local physicians. These travelers would come to town, register at a local hotel, advertise that they were specialists in certain types of illnesses, and treat those who flocked to their doors. Announcements of the arrival of such men were common in antebellum newspapers. In most cases they claimed to be well-trained physicians and therefore superior to the local practitioners who were most likely trained by apprenticeship.

In 1864 such a person came to Cleveland. Advertisements informed the public that Dr. J. F. Lawrence, "skilled oculist and aurist, has been working miracles in restoring lost and injured sight and hearing. He stays at the American House." On January 29, 1864, the *Cleveland Leader* reported to its readers that Lawrence had "skedaddled from the American House, cheating patients, landlord, and advertisers of $800." The following day, the *Leader* noted that "one month ago the city was honored by the distinguished arrival" of Dr. Lawrence, "at whose magical touch the blind saw and the deaf heard." "People visiting him and paying for his services," however, "were not benefitted by better eyes or ears." A reward was offered for his arrest.[23]

In addition to the heroic treatments that terrified the patients and the imposters whose actions cast aspersions on the entire medical profession, the physicians' economic status resulted in actions that further alienated the public. In most of the country, it was difficult to make a living by practicing medicine. This was especially the case in rural areas and among beginning physicians. It often was necessary for physicians to have some other means of support: "He must keep school (for which there is an opportunity in the winter), or till a piece of ground, or bring on a few goods (for the vending of which it is a good stand), or do something else in union with the practice of Physic."[24]

The economic realities of the practice of medicine led to a further deterioration of public support; the physician could hardly be respected when he appeared to be a local farmer with a sideline. Indeed, the status of the local physician might have been lower than that of the farmer, especially since the sturdy yeoman provided for his family by tilling the soil, whereas the physician had to raise crops because his chosen profession was so unprofitable.

When physicians united to improve their economic conditions, they further estranged themselves from the local populace. The better-trained physicians joined medical societies in the hope of improving conditions and advancing science. Soon they agreed to a "fee bill," a list of commonly accepted prices for services rendered. The intention was to prevent underbidding and to raise the economic level of the entire profession by charging reasonable fees that would enable the practitioner to support his family without having to moonlight.[25] The effect of the fee bill, however noble the intention, was to increase the cost of medical care by limiting economic competition between physicians. If it was bad enough to torture the public with heroic medicine, it was outrageous to raise the prices. In 1833, the physicians of Washington, D.C., signed a fee bill, which resulted in a series of meetings by enraged citizens and which ultimately led to an attempt to attract new practitioners who would not sign the fee bill.[26]

All the inadequacies of the orthodox medical profession combined to encourage the growth of unorthodox medical sects. The first important one was established in the early years of the nineteenth century by Samuel Thomson. Born and raised in rural New Hampshire, Thomson was almost totally uneducated. As a little boy he became friendly with "an old lady named Benton" who provided the medical care for the region, a medical care based on drugs she prepared from local plants and herbs. Thomson joined her on plant hunting expeditions and learned the medical properties of a great many plants. As he grew older he began to prescribe for his family. News of his ability spread through the area, and his neighbors called on him for treatment of their ailments. When his medical practice took too much time from his agricultural work, he abandoned farming and became a full-time physician.[27]

Thomson's system was based on his observation that four elements were present in all animal bodies: earth, air, fire and water, and cold. To Thomson, cold was the primary cause of illness. In order to cure disease, the practitioner had to "restore the natural heat" and clean the system of obstructions. This is similar to the old humoral theory, although undoubtedly Thomson was unaware of that fact. Thomson developed a list of botanical drugs that were combined with "steaming" the patient by a fire or on hot coals, treatments that certainly would "restore" the body's "natural heat."[28]

By 1809 Thomson had become an itinerant physician. He traveled through New England treating anyone who answered his advertisements. Local physicians were outraged that Thomson, who obviously was uneducated, was able to effect "great cures," and they were even more upset when some of their patients began to think more highly of Thomson than of the well-educated "scientific" practitioners. As a result, when Thomson lost a patient, Ezra Lovett, he found himself in trouble with the law. Lovett had a serious cold; Thomson had a fire built, ordered his patient to put his feet on a stove of hot coals, and had him drink hot coffee. When Lovett died, Thomson was charged with manslaughter by medical malpractice. He was locked in a Newburyport jail to await trial. His followers petitioned the Massachusetts Supreme Court, and Chief Justice Theophilus Parsons agreed to intervene and hear the case.

At the trial, witnesses testified that Thomson was completely ignorant of medical matters and that he called his drugs "ram-cats" and "well-my'gristle." The chief prosecution witness, a Doctor Howe, accused Thomson of poisoning his patient with lobelia, but he was unable to either identify or describe it. Manasseh Cutler, a well-known botanist, testified that the substance Thomson fed Lovett was a decoction of marsh rosemary and bark of bayberry bush, a harmless preparation. Others testified that Thomson's drugs were harmless and that he *had* effected "cures." After hearing the evidence the court found that the patient had died under the unskilled treatment of Thomson but that Thomson was innocent of manslaughter.[29]

In 1813 Thomson went to Washington, D.C., to secure a patent on his system of medical practice. When the patent was granted, he went into business. For twenty dollars anyone could purchase the "right" to heal himself and his family using the Thomsonian system and obtaining the necessary drugs from Thomson's company. Thomsonian "rights" were not licenses to practice medicine but only a guide to self-medication. Thomson declared that he wanted "to make every man his own physician." This was clearly in the American tradition of self-medication, especially in rural areas where there were too few trained physicians. Yet, in the first twenty years of the nineteenth century, self-medication was not as necessary as had previously been the case, especially in the settled regions of the nation. The little rural villages that once were secluded were becoming towns, and the towns were developing into cities, all with numerous physicians. As the frontier continued to move west, however, during the era of Manifest Destiny, there continued to be a ready market for guides to self-medication. Thomson followed a long line of men whose writings let every man be his own physician. In the eighteenth century William Buchan's *Domestic Medicine, or the Family Physician* played that role;[30] early in the nineteenth century James Ewell's *Planter's and Mariner's Medical Companion* served that purpose.[31]

Although Thomson never abandoned his original goal of helping every man be his own physician, many of those who had purchased "family rights" soon became practicing physicians. The historian cannot fault them for their decision to minister to friends and neighbors, especially when there was such popular suspicion of the orthodox practitioner and when their own treatments let nature take its course, quite the opposite of bloodletting and dosing with calomel.

Advocates of Thomsonianism believed that their system was far superior to heroic medicine, and they were willing to compete with the medical profession in the cities and towns. In 1828, for instance, Dr. George C. Shattuck wrote that as many as one-sixth of the people in Boston were attended by Thomsonian practitioners. Perhaps one explanation might be that the Thomsonians provided a familiar form of medicine for those who had migrated from rural to urban America, and of course it provided an alternative to bleeding, blistering, cupping, sweating, purging, and leeching. In 1842 the *Cleveland Herald* exclaimed that Thomson's great success "in establishing his steam and botanic practice of medicine, to some extent in nearly every portion of the United States, and in defiance, usually of ridicule and determined opposition, is pretty good evidence that his practice possesses no little efficacy as a curative process."[32]

The success of Thomsonianism was more related to the failings of orthodox medicine, however, than to the efficacy of cayenne pepper, for instance, as a curative agent. Perhaps one of William Lloyd Garrison's correspondents was correct when he wrote in 1838: "I would throw physic to the dogs and the cayenne pepper pot out of the window. The leech who put you on a course of cayenne," he exclaimed, "hath much to answer for."[33]

The success of Thomsonianism was also intimately related to the development of Jacksonian democracy in the period from 1820 to 1850. During that time there was a popular belief that the American common man could do anything and be anything; he had common sense that would enable him to be successful at anything he attempted. The common man insisted on his right to equal opportunity. That meant, of course, voting rights for white adult males, but it also meant an attack on all "monopolistic" practices. Laws that gave one man, one group, or one section an unfair advantage over others came in for a great deal of condemnation. It was natural for the medical license laws to be severely criticized during that time.

Those early laws established state medical societies and generally gave them the right to examine all applicants for licenses to practice medicine. Because the state medical societies were composed of relatively well-trained physicians and because the profession was having such a difficult time curing disease, it was commonly believed that they were hiding behind the law, that they were protecting themselves from competition with those more capable of success. In 1833 one newspaper declared that the law "can be of no possible benefit to the community at large." Rather, it "operates exclusively to the advantage of those at whose instance it has been brought into existence." The editor asserted that it was insulting "to the intelligence and discernment of our population to say that they are incapable of making a suitable selection of a physician, and that legislative enactments are requisite to prevent the people from inflicting an injury upon themselves."[34]

A brief glance at licensure in New York is necessary, at this point, to clarify the situation.[35] A battle developed between the allopaths, as the orthodox physicians were called, and the Thomsonians. The fast growth of botanical medicine was not only unscientific, but it constituted an economic threat to the medical profession. The orthodox practitioners rushed to the legislature for a law protecting themselves from "quacks." In 1806 the New York laws had provided for licensing by county medical societies, with the added provision that no unlicensed practitioner could sue for his fees. Then, in response to the lack of physicians in rural areas, the botanical physicians were exempted from the provisions of the law. When Thomsonianism developed in the state, the early law provided its practitioners with some protection. James Manley, a leading New York physician, was upset at the fact that the only penalty for practicing without a license was the inability to collect fees. He declared that it "punishes the *larceny,* while it acquits the *homicide!*"[36] The orthodox practitioners worked strenuously to convince the legislature of the need for truly restrictive laws against quackery.

In 1827 when the law was altered so that it no longer exempted the herbalists, a flood of petitions instigated by Thomsonians appealed on behalf of Jacksonian principles. Soon the Thomsonians were able to claim that more than 100,000 citizens demanded the total repeal of the medical license laws. The outcry resulted in the restoration in 1830 of the exemption of botanical practitioners. Now that the Thomsonians were experienced in political matters, the struggle continued. Finally, in 1844 the entire medical license law was repealed, making it legal for anyone to practice in the state, regardless of education or ability.

Similar battles took place in state after state. Almost all the medical license laws were repealed during the period from 1830 to 1850. In 1849 the newly established American Medical Association found that only New Jersey, Louisiana, and the District of Columbia still had regulatory laws.[37] At this point, the common man and the Thomsonians were clearly victorious. Their success may have ultimately resulted in an improvement in medical practice by forcing the orthodox physicians to moderate their treatments or else lose their patients to uneducated men who let nature do the healing.

It also resulted in chaos. In 1850 Lemuel Shattuck, the great pioneer in public health, declared in his *Report of the Sanitary Commission of Massachusetts* that "any one, male or female, learned or ignorant, an honest man or a knave, can assume the name of physician, and 'practice' upon any one, to cure or to kill, as either may happen, without accountability. It's a free country!"[38]

As early as 1838, David M. Reese, a New York physician and writer, gave an indication of what was to come. In his book, *The Humbugs of New York,* he declared that "the people regard it among their vested rights to buy and swallow such physick, as they in their sovereign will and pleasure shall determine; and in this free country, the democracy denounce all restrictions upon quackery as wicked monopolies for the benefit of physicians."[39]

Dr. Samuel Cartwright of Natchez, Mississippi, provided some statistics demonstrating a higher mortality rate after the repeal of his state's medical license law in 1833. As Cartwright exclaimed, as soon as it was legal to practice medicine, "cobblers left their lasts, blacksmiths their anvils, the barber threw aside his shaving brush, and even grey headed tailors jumped down from the board to become reformers in physic."[40] Being a "reformer" meant practicing medicine without the use of either the lancet or calomel.

While the battles over the license laws were being fought, several new medical sects joined the allopaths and the Thomsonians on the American scene. Each sought to attract patients and replace the heroic treatments of the orthodox practitioners. Dr. Wooster Beach was the main character in the faction whose members were known as eclectics. Beach was a graduate of New York's College of Physicians and Surgeons, but after several years of practice he abandoned the traditional orthodox treatments in favor of more moderate therapeutics. He developed a new system of medical practice, which substituted vegetable remedies for chemical ones. He called his sect the "American Reformed" system of practice, which took advantage of the intense nationalism pervading the country. In 1830, after establishing several Reformed societies in upstate New York, he decided to move west. At the same time, the Reform Medical Society of the

United States voted to establish a school on the Ohio River so that citizens near the frontier could benefit from "botanic medication." In 1832 Beach and Thomas V. Morrow established the school, located at Worthington, Ohio. It operated there until 1842, when it moved to Cincinnati and soon became known as the Eclectic Medical Institute.[41]

The eclectics emphasized that they were not tied to any one medical theory or practice but instead borrowed from the best of many systems. Although they were not averse to administering calomel or opium, for the most part they prescribed botanical remedies. Obviously they were closely related to the Thomsonians, but their specific connection with that group has yet to be proven. Traditionally historians have declared that eclectics were those botanical physicians who were dissatisfied with the low level of training given the Thomsonians and who thus developed medical colleges to train truly scientific "reformed" physicians. Evidence that this was the case seems to be lacking. In any event, the eclectics developed into a small but well-organized medical sect.

In the 1830s and 1840s another sect appeared on the scene. This was homeopathy, which soon became the leading and most influential irregular group. Homeopathy was developed in Europe by Samuel Christian Hahnemann, a German physician and an early experimental pharmacologist. Hahnemann's investigations and observations indicated that there were several laws of cure. The most important was *similia similibus curantur* (likes are cured by likes). Hahnemann became convinced that there was an inverse relationship between the size of the dose and the effect on the body. The more highly diluted the dose, the more effective it would be in combating disease. The physician, then, would try to prescribe a highly diluted dose of a drug, which, if given in a large dose to a healthy person, would produce the same set of symptoms.

The homeopathic physician devoted a great deal of time taking the patient's history in order to determine correctly the exact set of symptoms. Homeopathy proved to be extraordinarily successful in America. The scientific claims of homeopathy have never been subjected to objective unbiased examination; rather, they were cast aside by orthodox practitioners as being too ridiculous to merit serious study. How, they asked, could a dose as minute as one millionth of a gram be effective? Yet, the success of homeopathy could not be denied. Many orthodox physicians recognized this and cast aside the lancet and calomel in favor of the infinitesimal doses of homeopathy. It seemed evident that aside from any benefits that might be wrought by homeopathic treatment, the orthodox physicians were eliminating those patients who were too ill to endure heroic practices while the homeopaths were saving patients through supportive treatment.

Homeopathy did not really become significant in terms of numbers until after the 1850s, but by the 1870s and 1880s it was the largest and most influential sect. In terms of numbers, at its peak around the turn of the twentieth century, there was one homeopathic practitioner for every ten allopaths. The homeopaths tended to be congregated in the eastern states, especially New York, Massachusetts, and Pennsylvania, and in the cities with large immigrant populations. In Camden, New Jersey, for instance, in 1852 there were twenty-four regulars, two homeopaths, and one botanic. By 1872, there were thirty-two regulars, fourteen homeopaths, and five eclectics.[42]

It is clear that the development of the unorthodox sects and their appeal to the public were related to the shortcomings of the regular physicians. The orthodox medical profession was in decline, and the decline was accompanied by a change in public opinion over the years. In 1831 an article in the *North American Review* noted that "as a community, physicians are, more than most classes of men, made the butt of ridicule, and not unfrequently the subject of sweeping and unsparing censure." Every citizen considered his own physician to be above suspicion, possibly because of the low standard expected of such a maligned group of men.[43]

Dr. Edward Atwater has made an interesting study of the medical profession of Rochester from 1812 to 1860; his findings fit quite well into this analysis.[44] In the early years, the medical profession played a major role in municipal, religious, social, and economic affairs. As time passed, however, as the medical schools churned out more and more physicians of questionable ability, and with the irregulars practicing in larger numbers, the economic condition of the profession began to deteriorate. By 1860 physicians no longer played an influential role in civic affairs. The social and political role of the profession followed the economic condition, and the physician no longer had the widespread respect of the local community.

Worthington Hooker, a Yale professor and a leading Connecticut physician, analyzed the problems of the profession at the end of the 1840s, and he came to the conclusion that the problem was quackery and "the *spirit* of quackery" within the profession itself. Instead of being honorable men striving to save their patients, too many physicians sought reputations through dishonorable competition, advertising for patients, promising cures, giving testimonials to their successes, interfering with the work of other physicians, and so forth. Perhaps the physicians were following the example of the medical schools, which advertised in similar ways. Hooker even mentioned that some physicians gave gloomy prognostications to their patients in order to magnify their own importance if the patient survived and protect themselves from blame if the patient succumbed to the illness.[45]

The problems facing the profession were multifaceted, and the solution was complex. The first step to respectability had to be a transformation of American medical practice—the abandonment of the lancet and calomel in favor of more moderate therapeutics. As early as 1835, some leading physicians were starting to speak out against the abuse of the lancet and calomel. In that year, Jacob Bigelow read his pathfinding paper "On Self-Limited Diseases," which has been considered the first effective protest against heroic medicine in the United States.[46] Samuel Jackson continued the movement by declaring that the "least important part of the science . . . is the dosing of patients with medicine."[47]

By 1860 a great many physicians had abandoned heroic medicine; by 1870 bloodletting was not even being taught in America's medical schools.[48] This was a step in the direction of modern medicine and an even larger step in the return of the orthodox physician to respectability. The irregular practitioners could no longer appeal for patients on the basis of the terrifying allopathic treatments. They had to justify their own existence in terms of success and failure in curing patients at the precise time when the orthodox profession was breaking away from bloodletting and moving into the bacteriological age.

The second step toward true reform of the profession was in the revitalization of medical education. Worthington Hooker had declared that the solution to the problem facing the profession was through higher education of all physicians. "The lower the standard of education is among medical men," he declared, "the greater will be the number of ignorant pretenders who will gain admission into their ranks, and consequently the greater will be the prevalance of quackery in the profession, and of course in the community."[49]

There is no question that medical education was deficient. A great many physicians were practicing without any form of training except what they had learned as apprentices. In 1848, to give an example, more than one-fourth of the practitioners in Virginia had had no medical study other than through apprenticeship.[50] In addition to the large number of poorly educated physicians, the colleges were plagued with problems. As long as the schools competed for students by lowering requirements and reducing the length of the term, the trained physician was hardly worthy of public confidence. He may have been trained at an inferior school that had reduced standards in order to attract students. As long as these abuses continued, the public would continue to call on homeopaths, eclectics, and even Thomsonians to provide for their medical needs.

Notes

1. Benjamin Rush, *Medical Inquiries and Observations,* 3d ed. (Philadelphia, 1809), IV; 396, 411. Although the material in this chapter is by no means "new," it gives necessary information for those readers who are not familiar with American medical history.

2. William Cullen, *First Lines of the Practice of Physic* (New York, 1801), I: 37, 40, 67ff. See also the analysis in Lester S. King, *The Medical World of the Eighteenth Century* (Chicago, 1958), pp. 139ff.

3. See Nathan G. Goodman, *Benjamin Rush* (Philadelphia, 1934), pp. 229-254.

4. For material on the specific influence of Rush, see Goodman, *Benjamin Rush*, pp. 250-251, and Joseph I. Waring, "The Influence of Benjamin Rush on the Practice of Bleeding in South Carolina," *Bulletin of the History of Medicine* 35 (May-June 1961): 230-237.

5. Alexander Clendinen, comp., "Notes on the practice of Physic, from

the Lectures of Benjamin Rush, M.D., University of Pennsylvania, 1798,"
Toner Collection, Library of Congress.

6. See Charles S. Bryan, "Bloodletting in American Medicine, 1830-
1892," *Bulletin of the History of Medicine* 38 (November-December 1964):
516-529, and Martin Kaufman, *Homeopathy in America* (Baltimore, 1971),
pp. 3-6.

7. John B. Biddle, *Materia Medica for the Use of Students*, 8th ed.
(Philadelphia, 1878), pp. 17-19, 247-285. For a somewhat more detailed
description of the heroic treatments, see Kaufman, *Homeopathy in
America*, pp. 4-6. The reader should be aware that large-scale bleeding was
not limited to the United States. In France, Broussais and his followers bled
their patients as much as did American physicians.

8. Monteith diaries, 1808-1821, quoted in Fannie Anderson, *Doctors
Under Three Flags* (Detroit, 1951), pp. 138-140.

9. See William Prescott Papers, New York Public Library.

10. John P. Sheldon to Eliza Sheldon, Detroit, September 9, 1829, Sheldon Papers, Burton Historical Collection, Detroit Public Library.

11. Charles M. Bull to John Bull, Jr., Detroit, September 13, 1832,
November 25, 1832, C. M. Bull Papers, Burton Historical Collection.

12. Richard H. Shryock, *Medicine and Society in America: 1660-1860*
(Ithaca, New York, 1962) p. 131. See also Howard A. Kelly, *Cyclopedia of
American Medical Biography* (Philadelphia and London, 1912), I: 199-201.

13. Emily Mason to Catherine Mason Rowland, November 4, 1840, John
T. Mason Papers, Burton Historical Collection.

14. John Duffy, ed., *Rudolph Matas History of Medicine in Louisiana*
(Baton Rouge, 1962), II: 5.

15. *Western Journal of Medical and Physical Sciences* 7 (1833-1834): 187,
quoted in Duffy, *Rudolph Matas*, II: 5.

16. Hamilton County Medical Club, minutes, July 3, 1845, National
Library of Medicine, Bethesda, Maryland.

17. Duffy, *Rudolph Matas History of Medicine in Louisiana*, II: 12.

18. Quoted in "The Follies of the Faculty," *The United States Magazine,
and Democratic Review* 22 (April 1848): 360.

19. *Detroit Free Press,* December 23, 1859, from the "Digest Abstracted
by C. M. Burton," ms in Detroit Public Library.

20. James Harvey Young, "American Medical Quackery in the Age of the
Common Man," *Mississippi Valley Historical Review* 47 (1960-1961):
580-581.

21. Ibid., 586.

22. New Hampshire Medical Society, *Transactions, 1856* (Concord,
1856), 36, quoted in Young, *American Medical Quackery*, 582.

Heroic Age and Growth of the Irregulars

23. *Cleveland Leader,* January 15, 29, 30, 1864.

24. Stanley Griswold to James Witherell, May 28, 1809, quoted in Anderson, *Doctors Under Three Flags,* p. 90.

25. For instance, see the fee bill listed in Hamilton County Medical Club, minutes, May 4, 1844.

26. See Donald Konold, *History of American Medical Ethics, 1847-1912* (Madison, Wisconsin, 1962), p. 7.

27. For biographical information on Thomson, see Samuel Thomson, *A Narrative of the Life and Medical Discoveries of Samuel Thomson; Containing an Account of His System of Practice, and the Manner of Curing Disease with Vegetable Medicine, upon a Plan Entirely New,* 5th ed. (St. Clairsville, 1829), pp. 7-29.

28. See Frank G. Halstead, "A First-Hand Account of a Treatment by Thomsonian Medicine in the 1830's," *Bulletin of the History of Medicine* 10 (December 1941): 680-687. See also Philip D. Jordan, "The Secret Six, An Inquiry into the Basic Materia Medica of the Thomsonian System of Botanic Medicine," *Ohio State Archaeological and Historical Quarterly* 52 (October-December 1943): 347-355.

29. 6 Mass. 134; see also Thomson, *A Narrative,* pp. 72-84; Alexander Wilder, *History of Medicine* (New Sharon, Maine, 1901), pp. 457-459; William A. Purrington, "Manslaughter, Christian Science, and the Law," *Medical Record* 54 (November 26, 1898): 757.

30. William Buchan, *Domestic Medicine, or the Family Physician*(Edinburgh, 1769). It went through at least fourteen American editions.

31. James Ewell, *Planter's and Mariner's Medical Companion*(Philadelphia, 1807). For more on self-medication, see Anderson, *Doctors Under Three Flags,* pp. 100-101.

32. *Cleveland Herald,* May 28, 1842; George C. Shattuck to Jno. Homans, Boston, July 25, 1828, Massachusetts Historical Society, Boston.

33. E. Quincy to Garrison, Boston, June 14, 1838, Garrison Papers, Boston Public Library. Garrison often frequented unorthodox practitioners. See, for example, Garrison to Helen E. Garrison, Providence, May 5, 7, 1836, Garrison Papers.

34. *Cleveland Herald,* January 28, 1833.

35. For details on licensure in New York, see Joseph F. Kett, *The Formation of the American Medical Profession* (New Haven, 1968), pp. 12-22. An excellent study of the history of American medical licensing is Richard H. Shryock, *Medical Licensing in America, 1650-1965* (Baltimore, 1967).

36. James R. Manley, *Inaugural Address Delivered before the Medical Society of the State of New York* (New York, 1826), p. 19.

76 American Medical Education

37. See Henry B. Shafer, *The American Medical Profession, 1783-1850* (New York, 1936), pp. 211-214; William F. Norwood, *Medical Education in the United States Before the Civil War* (Philadelphia, 1944), p. 406; *Transactions of the American Medical Association, 1849* (Philadelphia, 1849), pp. 326-332.

38. Lemuel Shattuck, *Report of the Sanitary Commission of Massachusetts, 1850* (Cambridge, Massachusetts, 1948), p. 58, quoted in Young, "American Medical Quackery," *Mississippi Valley Historical Review* 47 (March 1961): 583.

39. David M. Reese, *The Humbugs of New York* (New York, 1838), p. 124.

40. Samuel A. Cartwright, "Remarks on Statistical Medicine, Contrasting the Result of the Empirical with the Regular Practice of Physic, in Natchez," *Western Journal of Medicine and Surgery* 2 (July 1840): 3.

41. For more on eclectics, see Vincent Millasich, "Eclecticism and Its Origin," *California Eclectic Medical Journal* 6 (December 1913): 299-301; Mason M. Miles, "Medical Reform," *Chicago Medical Times* 13 (September 1881): 265-267; A. H. Collins, "Principles and Progress of the Eclectic School of Medicine," *National Eclectic Medical Association Quarterly* 7 (March 1916): 267-276. For a history of the eclectic colleges, see Frederick C. Waite, "American Sectarian Medical Colleges before the Civil War," *Bulletin of the History of Medicine* 19 (February 1946): 148-166.

42. E. L. B. Godfrey, *History of the Medical Profession of Camden County* (Philadelphia, 1896), pp. 32-33, 113. For additional information on the history of homeopathy, see Kaufman, *Homeopathy in America.* For more on the place of eclectics in American medicine, see Ronald L. Numbers, "The Making of an Eclectic Physician: Joseph M. McElhinney and the Eclectic Medical Institute of Cincinnati," *Bulletin of the History of Medicine* 47 (March-April 1973): 155-166.

43. "Character and Abuses of the Medical Profession," *North American Review* 32 (April 1831): 368-369.

44. Edward Atwater, "The Medical Profession in a New Society: Rochester, New York (1811-1860)," *Bulletin of the History of Medicine* 47 (May-June 1973): 221-235.

45. Worthington Hooker, *Physician and Patient* (New York, 1849), 250-253.

46. Jacob Bigelow, *Nature in Disease* (Boston, 1854), pp. 1-58. See also Richard Shryock, *Medicine and Society in America* (New York, 1960), pp. 131-132.

47. Address to Medical Graduates, University of Pennsylvania, 1840, quoted in Shryock, *Medicine and Society in America,* p. 131.

48. See Bryan, "Bloodletting."

49. Hooker, *Physician and Patient,* pp. 250-253.

50. *Transactions of the American Medical Association, 1848* (Philadelphia, 1848), pp. 359-360.

5

The Beginning of Reform, 1825-1846

Almost as soon as physicians diagnosed the problems of their profession, they began to prescribe remedies, all of which centered on the colleges. It was inevitable that the conflict between the schools and the state medical societies was to play a major role in the debates that developed. After all, the proliferation of the colleges and the reduction of their standards decreased the quality of medical practice and helped to destroy the prestige of the profession. That was detrimental to the societies but financially beneficial to the colleges. The medical reformers, then, belonged to either of two groups. They were conscientious educators who were upset at the results of the competition between colleges, or they were physicians who blamed the educators for the problems facing the entire medical profession.

The first significant attempt at reform came as early as 1825 when the Vermont State Medical Society proposed an increase in requirements for degrees and licenses. In order to improve the quality of medical care, the members of the society suggested that no one be graduated or licensed to practice medicine unless he had taken at least one course of medical lectures.[1] The Vermont society also proposed that the colleges confer the bachelor's degree in medicine, with the doctorate being granted only to those who especially merited it after seven years of medical practice and advanced study. Finally, the Vermont physicians decided to send a circular letter to other state medical societies and colleges in the hope that they could encourage a far-reaching reform.

The result was a great deal of discussion on the merits of the Vermont plan to reform medical education. On October 4, 1826, the Counsellors of the Massachusetts Medical Society established a committee consisting of John Collins Warren, John Dixwell, and George Hayward to study the Vermont proposal and make recommendations.[2] One month later the committee reported it was in favor of medical reform, and it commented on the specific proposals of the Vermont society. The committee agreed with the New Hampshire Medical Society, which had suggested that two courses of lectures, rather than one, be required for graduation and for licensing.[3]

Warren, Dixwell, and Hayward were opposed to the suggestion that the bachelor's degree be reinstituted. They argued that it was contrary to precedent; the bachelor's degree had been abandoned in favor of the doctorate. They predicted, quite correctly, that very few candidates would return for an advanced degree. "In the earlier years of the Medical Institution of Harvard University," they said, not only was the doctor's degree "rarely sought," but few bachelor's degrees were conferred because students attended "some other seminary where the requirements were less complex." Finally the committee, and ultimately the society, proposed that a convention of medical colleges and societies be held "in some central place."[4] It was determined to hold that convention at Northampton, Massachusetts, in June 1827. The stage was set for a thorough discussion of the problems of medical education by delegates of the societies and colleges of New England.

The medical societies of Maine, New Hampshire, Vermont, Massachusetts, and Connecticut sent delegates to the Northampton convention, and representatives from Bowdoin, Brown, Dartmouth, Harvard, and the Berkshire Medical Institution also attended. The specifics of their discussions seem to be lost, but they recorded their conclusions. They agreed that it was necessary to improve the preliminary education of medical students, and they decided that every candidate for a medical license or degree should either hold a bachelor of arts degree or give evidence of a good education, including a knowledge of Latin, geometry, and natural philosophy.[5]

The delegates decided that every applicant for a medical license should have to present evidence that he had studied medicine for at least three years. Those applicants who were not college graduates would be required to study four years with a licensed practitioner. They determined that "no student shall be allowed to absent himself from his studies more than six weeks in any one year of his professional pupilage," a direct response to the fact that many medical students farmed, taught school, or kept a store for a good part of the year.

They decided that every candidate for a medical license examination must be over the age of twenty-one, must have taken at least one full course of medical lectures, and must be able to pass an examination in anatomy, physiology, surgery, theory and practice of medicine, materia medica, chemistry, and midwifery, as well as write and defend a dissertation. These requirements, if enforced, would have prevented all but a select few from entering the medical profession. Of course, to a large extent the discussion was strictly academic; the impulse of Jacksonian democracy was resulting in the abandonment of medical license laws and the reduction of the powers of medical societies. In a very short time, these requirements could not possibly have been enforced. Nevertheless the convention delegates then discussed the requirements for degrees. They decided that every candidate for a medical degree must take two full courses of lectures and be able to pass an examination on the same medical subjects required of all licensed practitioners, along with tests on botany and medical jurisprudence.

The delegates proposed that the requirements on preliminary education go into effect on July 4, 1829. They thus would not penalize those students already enrolled in the various colleges, and they would give apprentices two years' notice that they would be expected to demonstrate evidence of a good education, with a knowledge of Latin, geometry, and natural philosophy.

Finally, the convention decided to establish the Association of Medical Societies and Institutions to meet periodically and develop mutually acceptable reforms, which would raise the caliber of the profession through improvements in medical education. In order to be a member of the association, medical societies and colleges had to accept the requirements adopted at the Northampton convention. A central committee, consisting of James Jackson of Harvard, James P. Chaplin of the Massachusetts Medical Society, and John C. Warren of Boston, was elected to plan future meetings and to handle the communications required in maintaining the cordial relations developed at the first meeting.

When the delegates returned to their colleges and societies, discussion developed on the feasibility of instituting such far-reaching changes. The medical societies of Maine and Vermont and the medical schools at Bowdoin, Dartmouth, Brown, and the University of Vermont gave their unqualified support to the proposals. The medical societies of New Hampshire and Massachusetts approved the suggestions but with certain changes. The New Hampshire society insisted that students be allowed to be employed in some other occupation, but not for more than sixteen weeks in any one year. Undoubtedly this was a response to the fact that rural physicians had apprentices who were expected by their parents to help out on the farm.[6]

The Massachusetts Medical Society and Harvard College insisted that every candidate for a license, as well as for a degree, attend two courses of lectures, pass an examination, and present and defend a medical dissertation. In addition, they wanted it understood that adoption of the reforms did not prevent any college or society from demanding additional qualifications for degrees or licenses.[7]

It would have been too much to expect the Northampton convention to bring about a real and lasting reform of medical education. The colleges and the societies had totally opposite interests. The colleges could not be expected to adopt reforms that might encourage students to attend schools that did not accept those reforms, especially when medical schools depended upon student fees for their existence. The societies, on the other hand, wanted to protect their right of licensure at a time when the states were repealing the medical license laws and when it could clearly be foreseen that in the near future anyone could practice medicine without any examination and, indeed, without any qualifications.

The physicians who were members of the various medical societies apparently saw licensure as the way to limit entrance into the profession at the time when physicians were starting to believe that the profession was overpopulated. The delegates from the societies, then, wanted to develop stringent rules and regulations to ensure that only qualified individuals entered medical practice. The colleges, on the other hand, could not accept those rules unless they all accepted the same regulations and unless it could be determined that the rules would not adversely affect enrollment and income at the colleges. The necessary cooperation, however, was lacking. According to Whitfield Bell, Yale College was the only school to abide by the recommendations of the Northampton convention. When no other college increased its requirements and raised its standards, Yale faced the real possibility of decreased enrollments. As a result, the faculty was forced to return to its previous, though inadequate, system of medical education.[8]

The failings of the convention can also be seen, to some extent, in the way Harvard's medical faculty changed requirements after the 1827 meeting. From 1827 to 1833 it made no alterations. In October 1833 the faculty voted that students who were not college graduates be examined in natural philosophy and Latin before being examined in the various medical branches. This came four years after the Northampton reforms were to go into effect. Then, in May 1840, the faculty voted to dispense with examinations in natural philosophy and Latin "in those cases in which the student furnishes certificates of competent knowledge in these branches." In addition, even though the Harvard faculty had agreed with the state medical society in demanding that candidates for both degrees and licenses attend two full courses of lectures, it was not until May 1841 that that was required for graduation from Harvard.[9]

By the early 1830s, it was obvious that the Northampton convention was a failure. In spite of all the discussion, very little reform of medical education resulted, and conditions were continuing to deteriorate throughout the nation; reform was needed more than ever. Not only had the schools continued to proliferate, but by then the movement to repeal the medical license laws was in full swing.

In 1834 and 1835, events in Georgia were to encourage a renewed demand for a medical convention. Recognizing the difficulties with the existing system of medical education, the faculty of the Medical

College of Georgia lengthened its term to six months and rearranged the entire program of medical training. In order to provide a better atmosphere for learning, the daily number of lectures was reduced to three or four. The afternoons were to be devoted to dissection and the evenings to reading. As could well be expected, many students transferred to colleges that expected less of the students. Joseph Eve, the professor of therapeutics and materia medica, declared that the students wanted to graduate "with as little exertion as possible—content to practice . . . as a mere *trade,* or at most to attain, to an ignoble mediocrity," which he said was "scarcely less disgraceful than professed empiricism."[10]

The faculty had hoped to be able to maintain high standards, but with so few students the college could barely remain in operation. As a result, the faculty decided to call a national convention of medical colleges to develop uniform standards that would enable *all* the colleges to advance together. The convention was scheduled to be held in May 1836 in Washington, D.C., but unfortunately not one college sent delegates. The attempt of the Medical College of Georgia was a total failure.[11]

At the same time a movement was developing to raise standards in the state of Ohio. In June 1834, William M. Awl of Columbus started the movement when he sent a circular to "all Scientific Practitioners" of medicine and surgery in Ohio calling for a convention. He specifically stated that medical reform was necessary in order to rectify "the great depression of character . . . which unhappily prevail[s]" in the medical profession. Awl's letter indicated that he envisioned possible solutions to various problems facing the medical profession, among them the regulation of "professional etiquette," the establishment of state and local medical societies, support of a journal, and ways to ensure the "convenient supply of the Leech." In addition to such medical reforms, Awl was fully committed to the general reform movement in American society. He expected the convention to discuss also the need to erect asylums "for the reception of Lunatics and the instruction of the Blind," as well as the "promotion of the temperance cause."[12]

Awl's letter provoked a fairly good response from Ohio's physicians, possibly because he had suggested so many areas of reform that it appealed to a great many individuals. On January 5, 1835, the Ohio

convention of physicians began its deliberations. Almost immediately a committee was established to report on "the means of
improving the state of medical education in Ohio." Daniel Drake,
Landon C. Rives, Silas Reed, and Awl served on this committee. Two
schools were represented on the committee: Drake was affiliated
with the Medical College of Ohio and Rives was professor of obstetrics in the medical department of Cincinnati College.[13]

The committee reported that there were a number of "radical
defects" in the existing system of medical education, defects that if
not corrected "must ultimately annihilate whatever of respectability
remains to the profession." It suggested increasing the standards of
preliminary education and assuring that physicians serving as preceptors were well prepared. Most important, the committee proposed that the colleges unite in order to lengthen sessions and elevate
standards. The convention adopted the committee report and
adjourned after resolving to hold a second convention three years
later in January 1838.[14] The physicians who were present at the
convention obviously and somewhat naively hoped that they had
solved the problem by informing colleges of the ways to improve
medical education. Presumably the colleges would reform themselves, thus improving the quality of medical practice in the state.

Unfortunately, it seems that the colleges totally ignored the convention recommendations. The two delegates from the Medical College of Ohio, for instance, reported simply that the visit to Columbus
was "useful," and happily noted that "no attack had been made on the
College."[15] Since the convention would not reconvene until 1838,
the college took no action to remedy its defects.

It was naive to expect the colleges to reform themselves. After all,
many of them had been established as a result of professional
jealousy, and each of them was engaged in ruthless competition with
other colleges. It would have taken a combination of Solomon-like
wisdom and a direct threat to the survival of the schools to bring
about the harmony necessary for a lasting reform of medical education.

When the Ohio medical convention reconvened in 1838, Daniel
Drake's committee "on the causes which contribute to depress the
science, dignity and influence" of the profession reported that there
had been little change over the past three years. The committee

reported that the benches at the medical colleges were filled with men who were deficient not only in classical training but also "in a common English education." One basic problem it noted was that a number of young men began medical practice before they were qualified to do so. It was common for men in the South and West to begin practicing "after a brief period of private pupilage, without visiting any medical school," or after one course of lectures.[16]

Drake's committee reported that the "science, dignity and influence" of the profession were low because of the insufficient compensation derived from medical practice. There were so many "physicians" that the fees had to be reduced. Indeed the average physician could not possibly afford an adequate library or other apparatus he might need in his work. A large number of physicians were so destitute, according to the report, that they had to add "some other business to the practice of medicine." Because compensation was so low the best students decided to enter the other professions. At the same time, the inadequate compensation discouraged future physicians from devoting a great deal of time to preparing for their future. The inevitable result was a mass of poorly prepared practitioners.[17]

Another committee described the defects in medical education. This committee, consisting of J. P. Kirtland, Daniel J. M. Peixotto, and the ever-present Daniel Drake, recommended that the courses of lectures be extended by one month and that the pupils be required to remain to the end of the session rather than leaving earlier, as often was the case. It also suggested that more professors be added to the various faculties; most schools had too few instructors to cover the realm of medical science. Drake's committee proposed that there be a graded curriculum. Each student should take anatomy, physiology, chemistry, and pharmacy in the first year, while the second year would be devoted to pathology, anatomy, therapeutics, medical practice, surgery, and obstetrics. In this way, inadequately prepared students would no longer be forced to take all the courses at the same time, even though some courses presupposed a depth of knowledge and experience lacking in so many students. Finally, the committee reported that the quality of the typical student was too low. It recommended increased standards of preliminary education to ensure that the students benefit from their medical training. Furthermore, it suggested that no student be graduated unless he was over twenty-one and that all graduates show evidence of having completed at least four years of medical study, combining college work and apprenticeship.

The committee proposed to call a convention of all the American colleges, to provide "a simultaneous co-operative effort" to improve the quality of medical education, and it suggested that notice be sent to all the medical institutions in the United States so that reform would not be restricted to one state or one area. In that way, they might reduce the possibility of failure; with a nationwide reform students could not enroll at a low standard school.[18] The Ohio convention adopted the committee report, but once again there was no mad rush to reform medical education.

At this point, the scene shifted from Ohio to New Hampshire. In June 1838 the New Hampshire Medical Society noted the problems facing the profession and voted to recommend an annual convention to meet starting in 1840. Notice was sent to the *Boston Medical and Surgical Journal* and the *American Journal of the Medical Sciences,* but the New Hampshire attempt at reform fell on deaf ears, as had the earlier attempt sponsored by the faculty of the Medical College of Georgia.[19]

Nevertheless virtually every state medical society began to discuss the problems of the profession, especially when the power to license was eliminated by the repeal of the state laws. Every discussion ultimately centered on problems in medical education. On February 7, 1839, the Medical Society of the State of New York held its discussion, which resulted in the only continuing drive for reform. During the debate, John McCall of Utica offered a resolution calling for a convention to be held in Philadelphia in 1840. McCall's motion was adopted with the provision that each society send three delegates and each college send one delegate.[20] Undoubtedly this was intended to ensure that the colleges could be outvoted and that the societies would be able to make reforms even if the professors were opposed to them.

When the proposed date for the convention arrived, May 12, 1840, not one school sent a delegate; Robley Dunglison of the Jefferson Medical College declared that the intended birth of American medical reform turned out to be "an abortion." Daniel Drake was upset at the failure, and he complained that "the time for reform has assuredly arrived—the cry for it comes up from all parts of the country." In spite of that "cry" for reform, only a handful of delegates appeared for the convention, all from New Hampshire, New York, and Ohio.[21]

In January 1843 Dean Thomas D. Mitchell of Transylvania University sent letters to inform the medical schools of the western states that the Transylvania faculty had discussed ways to elevate the quality of medical education in the region and had proposed that the area schools meet to work out some mutually agreeable arrangement. When the letter arrived at the Medical College of Ohio, it was submitted to a faculty committee, which decided that if the other schools agreed to three rules, it would be willing to raise its standards. First, the colleges would assure that no one graduate who had not studied medicine for three full years, including two full courses of medical lectures. Second, the schools would abolish the practice of giving credit simply on possession of lecture tickets. Finally, the colleges would refrain from graduating experienced practitioners on the basis of one course of lectures. This was unacceptable to Transylvania, and Mitchell notified the Medical College of Ohio that "it is inexpedient to make any general arrangement, respecting the government of Medical Schools."[22]

The New York society, however, continued to discuss the need for reform. In 1844 it resolved that the four-month term was too short for adequate lectures on all the branches of medicine and that the standards of preliminary and medical education were too low to ensure the graduation of qualified physicians. The following year the discussion shifted to the possibility of raising standards in New York. Nathan Smith Davis, who was soon to become the leader of the drive to reform medical education, suggested that students be required to pass examinations before graduation and before licensing. His recommendation was opposed by delegates who feared that high standards in one state would only raise the income of out-of-state schools by driving students away from the New York colleges. When everyone present seemed to agree that it would be self-defeating for New York to unilaterally increase standards, Alden March, a founder of Albany Medical College, suggested to Davis that there was a solution: a national medical convention. Davis moved that a meeting to reform medical education be held in New York City in May 1846.[23]

Once again, the call for a convention did not provoke an enthusiastic response. Professors at the Philadelphia colleges were convinced that the convention was intended to advertise the New York schools rather than to bring about the needed reforms in medical education. At this point, Martyn Paine of the New York University Medical School published a condemnation of the New York society for calling such a meeting. In his *Defence of the Medical Profession of the United States,* Paine declared that if the standards of education were to be raised to European standards, "quackery will reign almost universal from one end of the continent to the other." He predicted that if standards were increased, the medical schools would drive "most of their aspirants into more humble channels, or into the walks of empiricism." If not for "an early harvest" of physicians, he said, the profession would "soon be overrun with weeds."[24]

Paine complained that the move to reform medical education had "an *aristocratic* feature." "It is oppression towards the poor, for the sake of crippling the principal Medical Colleges." He declared that successful medical reform would limit the field "to the few who may spring from families of wealth," those who were able to afford an adequate preliminary education and a lengthy course of studies. Paine seemed most upset at the fact that in his enthusiasm for medical reform, Davis had declared in the *New York Journal of Medicine* that 99 percent of the American physicians were deficient in education and that many could not even write their own names.[25]

Paine had voiced similar sentiments back in 1843. In an introductory address to his class at the University of New York, he said that Americans have always sought the cheapest and fastest solution to every problem. As a result, any attempt to reform medical education would fail, as it would encourage students to practice medicine before they were adequately prepared. Interestingly, Paine's school practiced what he preached; at least Alfred Stillé, a leading Philadelphia physician, believed that to be the case. He wrote in a letter to Harvard's George C. Shattuck that it was strange that "students who resort to New York should prefer that rotten & disgraceful concern to the dignified and meritorious" College of Physicians and Surgeons. Stillé declared: "Heaven only knows what is to become of all the Doctors ground, or rather bolted, out of the innumerable mills from Maine to Texas. They should be sent as pioneers to Oregon."[26]

When Robert M. Huston of the Jefferson Medical College read Paine's *Defence of the Profession,* he realized that the call for a convention was not intended to advertise the medical schools of New York, as Paine was clearly speaking for one of the New York schools. Rather, Huston recognized, it was a serious attempt to bring about reform of medical education. He used his influence to convince the Philadelphia County Medical Society to send twelve delegates to the national convention, and the Philadelphia colleges decided to send delegates. When the convention finally met on May 5, 1846, there were 119 delegates from sixteen states.[27]

As the "national medical convention" came to order, Gunning Bedford of New York University moved that the session begin by adjourning. His motion was seconded by G. S. Pattison, also of New York University. One can only imagine the feelings of those who had travelled some distance in the hope of participating in a real reform of medical education when Bedford made his motion, which would have ended the convention and the hope of reform. The motion lost by a vote of seventy-four to two. Then N. S. Davis moved that a committee be established to discuss the problems of medical education and to make recommendations for possible solutions. On the following day, May 6, the committee, which included Davis and Alden March, reported a series of resolutions. It recommended that the convention be the nucleus of a national medical association to allow for a continuing improvement of American medicine. Then it proposed that "a uniform and elevated standard of requirements . . . be adopted by all the Medical Schools in the United States" and that a seven-man committee be appointed to make specific recommendations for the elevation of standards. The resolution was adopted and the committee appointed, including John Cullen of the Medical College of Virginia, Austin Flint of the University of Buffalo, Robert W. Haxall of Richmond, George W. Norris of Philadelphia, Samuel A. Patteson of Manchester, Virginia, Joseph Perkins of the Castleton Medical College, and Joel A. Wing of Albany.[28]

Davis' committee then proposed that before admission to medical school, all students should "have acquired a suitable preliminary education," and it recommended that a seven-man committee be established to make specific recommendations on the type of preliminary education necessary to upgrade the entire profession. When this was adopted, the committee was appointed, including Washington Atlee of Pennsylvania College, D. T. Brainard of New London, Lewis P. Bush and James W. Thomson of Wilmington, Delaware, James Couper of Newcastle, Delaware, Alden March of the Albany Medical College, and Edward Mead of the Illinois Medical College.[29]

Next, Dr. O. S. Bartles of New York City completely divided the convention by moving "that the Union of the business of *Teaching* and Licensing in the same hands is wrong in principle and liable to great abuse in practice" and that the power to license "should be restricted to one Board in each State, composed in fair proportion of representatives from its Medical Colleges and the Profession at Large, and the pay for whose services as Examiners should in no degree depend on the number licensed by them." After a debate on the relationship between the societies and the colleges, the proposal was referred to a special committee to report the following year. The committee included Rufus Blakeman of Fairfield, Connecticut, Thomas Cock of New York City, John Cullen of the Medical College of Virginia, John W. Francis and James R. Manley of New York City, James McNaughton of the Albany Medical College, and Isaac Parrish of Philadelphia.[30]

Having provided the groundwork for the establishment of what became the American Medical Association and having developed procedures for a thorough examination of the problems of medical education, the delegates to the first national medical convention voted to adjourn. It was a historical gathering in New York City, one that was to play a major role in professionalizing American medicine. The question of successfully reforming medical education and uplifting the prestige of the profession, however, was to be delayed for at least one more year, awaiting the recommendations of the committees established at the first convention. Although ten states had no representation and only about one-third of the colleges sent delegates, it was a promising step in the direction of reform.[31]

Notes

1. For a discussion on events from Vermont to the national convention in 1846, see Byron Stookey, "Origins of the First National Medical Convention: 1826-1846," *Journal of the American Medical Association* 177 (July 15, 1961): 123ff; Vermont Medical Society, minutes, October 14, 1825, Wilbur Collection, Bailey Library, University of Vermont, Burlington, Vermont.

2. Massachusetts Medical Society, proceedings of the counsellors, October 4, 1826, in *Medical Communications* (Boston, 1826), IV: 21ff.

3. Ibid., November 7, 1826.

4. Ibid.

5. The following description of the convention is based upon *Proceedings of a Convention of Medical Delegates, Held at Northampton (June 20, 1827)* (Boston, 1827).

6. *Boston Medical and Surgical Journal* 1 (October 7, 1828): 538-40.

7. Ibid., (June 24, 1828): 301-302. See also Minute Book of the Harvard Medical Faculty, January 10, 1827, August 17, 1827, Countway Library, Harvard University.

8. Whitfield Bell, Jr., "The Medical Institution of Yale College, 1810-1885," *Yale Journal of Biology and Medicine* 33 (December 1960): 175. For details on the changes in the Yale program, see *Proceedings of the Connecticut Medical Society, 1792-1829*, minutes, May 13, 14, 1829; *Proceedings of the President and Fellows of the Connecticut Medical Society, at their Annual Convention in May, 1830* (Hartford, 1830), p. 15; *Proceedings of the President and Fellows of the Connecticut Medical Society in Convention May, 1834* (New Haven, 1834), pp. 14-15.

9. Harvard Medical faculty, minutes, October 5, 1833, May 2, 1840, May 29, 1841.

10. Joseph A. Eve, "Medical Education," *Southern Medical and Surgical Journal* (Augusta, Georgia) 1 (September 1836): 216-219.

11. Ibid., 220-226; N. S. Davis, *History of the American Medical Association, from Its Organization up to January, 1855* (Philadelphia, 1855), pp. 20-21.

12. *Journal of the Proceedings of a Convention of Physicians of Ohio* (Cincinnati, 1835), p. 4.

13. Ibid., p. 6. Drake was interested in the general reform movement in American society. See the collection held by the Cincinnati General Hospital Library.

14. Ibid., pp. 20-24.

15. Medical College of Ohio faculty, minutes, January 10, 1835, Archives

of Medical History, University of Cincinnati Library.

16. *Journal of the Proceedings of the Medical Convention of Ohio* (Cincinnati, 1838), pp. 9-14.

17. Ibid.

18. Ibid., p. 17. See also *Western Journal of Medicine and Surgery*, 1 (May 31, 1840): 366-368.

19. *American Journal of the Medical Sciences* 23 (November 1838): 264.

20. See *Western Journal of Medicine and Surgery* 1: 366-368; Davis, *History of the A. M. A.*, pp. 20-21; *Proceedings of the Third Medical Convention of Ohio* (Cleveland, 1839), pp. 43-46.

21. Davis, *History of the AMA*, pp. 20-21; *Western Journal of Medicine and Surgery* 1: 366-368.

22. Medical College of Ohio, faculty, minutes, January 18, January 28, February 25, and March 11, 1843.

23. Davis, *History of the AMA*, pp. 22-24. For a biography of Davis, see I. N. Danforth, *Life of Nathan Smith Davis* (Chicago, 1907), and Otto F. Kampmeier, "Nathan Smith Davis, 1817-1904: A Biographical Essay," *Journal of Medical Education* 34 (May 1959): 496-508.

24. Martyn Paine, *A Defence of the Medical Profession of the United States*, 8th ed. (New York, 1846), pp. 8-9.

25. Ibid., pp. 15-16.

26. Martyn Paine, "A Lecture on the Improvement of Medical Education in the United States," *New York Journal of Medicine* 1 (November 1843): 367-378; Alfred Stillé to George C. Shattuck, Philadelphia, March 26, 1844, Shattuck Papers, Massachusetts Historical Society.

27. Davis, *History of the AMA*, pp. 30-32.

28. *Proceedings of the National Medical Conventions Held in New York, May, 1846, and in Philadelphia, May, 1847*(Philadelphia, 1847), pp. 15-17.

29. Ibid.

30. Ibid., p. 19.

31. Davis, *History of the AMA*, p. 37. States with no representation were Alabama, Kentucky, Louisiana, Maine, Missouri, Michigan, North Carolina, Ohio, South Carolina, and Texas, according to Davis' account.

6

The American
Medical Association,
1847-1860

During the next year, the various committees were hard at work. They did a great deal of research, sent questionnaires to the colleges and to other interested parties, and developed their recommendations. When the National Medical Convention reconvened in Philadelphia in 1847, the committees were prepared to submit their reports.

The committee on "uniform and elevated standards or requirements" was first on the agenda. Its report began on a conciliatory note; medicine, it noted, had been better taught in the past twenty or twenty-five years than ever before, but much more could be done to improve the quality of medical teaching. Then it declared, quite correctly, that "the large number of Medical Colleges throughout the country, and the facility with which the degree is obtained, have exerted a most pernicious influence." Medical education had declined to such an extent that "each returning spring lets loose upon the community some twelve or thirteen hundred graduates" to cure or to kill. The committee placed a good part of the blame on the preceptorial system. So many preceptors had accepted as apprentices students who were totally unprepared for medical practice that "often has it been asserted, that the Veriest dolts possessed intellect sufficient for the study of medicine."[1]

The committee reported that it had sent questionnaires to every American college to learn exactly what the standards were and to be able to develop a proposal that would raise standards to the level of the better schools. It received nineteen replies, representing slightly more than half of the schools. The results indicated a great variation among the colleges. The number of professors varied from three to eight; the term extended from three months in some schools to eight months in others; clinical instruction was required in twelve colleges and not in seven; dissection was required in five schools but only recommended in fourteen.[2]

The committee made its specific proposals in the form of ten recommendations. If they were adopted, the committee believed that medical education would be advanced to such an extent that every medical graduate would be fully qualified to practice medicine. The recommendations included lengthening the term to six months and requiring graduates to take two courses of lectures and to present evidence of having completed an apprenticeship with a qualified preceptor. In addition, the committee suggested that there be seven professors in each college providing instruction in seven branches of medical science: theory and practice of medicine, principles and practice of surgery, general and special anatomy, physiology and pathology, materia medica, therapeutics and pharmacy, midwifery and the diseases of women and children, and chemistry and medical jurisprudence. Finally it recommended that each student be required to devote three months to anatomical dissection, that preceptors provide clinical instruction, and that the colleges require hospital practice.[3] The delegates to the national convention adopted the committee report.

The committee on the preliminary education of students then submitted its report. It had sent queries to the thirty-one colleges but received only six replies—from Albany Medical College, New York's College of Physicians and Surgeons, Dartmouth, Ohio Medical College, University of Pennsylvania, and Yale. The committee decided that the chief responsibility for training young doctors must rest with the preceptors; they were the ones who encouraged young men to enter the profession and they provided the early medical training. Nevertheless, it stated, the colleges had an obligation to ascertain that students were well-enough prepared to benefit from medical education. The committee called for uniform standards of preliminary education, neither too low nor too high. It wanted to exclude those who were obviously incapable of becoming successful practitioners, without eliminating those "meritorious young men of limited means and opportunities." The committee said that the preceptor must determine the quality of the preliminary education of his students and certify to it. The colleges should require each student to submit that certificate and publish the names of the preceptors. Presumably a preceptor would not certify the education of a student who might prove to be one of those "veriest dolts" mentioned by the first committee if he knew that his action would become common knowledge. This report was also adopted by the delegates.[4]

Finally, the reports were submitted by the committee established to report on Dr. Bartles' motion on the control of licensing. The committee members could not come to a consensus, so they submitted two reports. The majority (Cock, Francis, Manley, and Parrish) reported that when the colleges were first given the power to award degrees, which in effect were licenses to practice medicine, it was a beneficial development. At that time, there were few trained physicians, and the best talent was concentrated in a few colleges. Since then, the proliferation of the colleges and the ensuing competition had produced some "very defective schools," which "live and flourish, and even outstrip the more competent." The committee declared that the abuses would continue until the legislatures took greater care in granting charters to medical colleges or until the profession could unite to develop higher standards. The report insisted that the profession demand participation in the licensing of physicians.[5]

It was a weak and ineffectual report, and generally a correct one considering the circumstances. Perhaps it should be explained at this point that originally the colleges did not have anything resembling the "licensing power" discussed by the members of the committee. The state medical societies had examined applicants for medical licenses, and the colleges tried to prepare students for the examinations. When the states repealed their licensing laws during the

Jacksonian period, that in effect gave the colleges "licensing power."
The schools were already authorized to grant degrees, and in the
absence of restrictive legislation, possession of a doctorate was tantamount to a medical license, giving the doctor a competitive advantage over those whose training was solely through apprenticeship.
Without help from the legislatures, the "licensing power" could not
possibly be removed from the colleges and returned to the profession
at large. The leaders of the American medical profession could only
hope to publicize the situation and work toward professional unity,
which might convince the colleges to accept the needed reforms.

The minority (Cock and McNaughton) agreed that abuses did exist,
but they did not believe that it was wrong in principle to mix teaching
and licensing. The professors, they said, were in the best position to
determine the qualifications of their own students. Cock and
McNaughton proposed that medical license examinations be
administered by boards consisting of professors and members of the
profession at large, "not for the purpose of embarrassing the faculty
or candidates, but . . . to relieve the institutions themselves" of
censure.[6]

After some debate, the delegates decided to table both reports to
the committee on medical education, where they were allowed to die
a natural death. In any case, licensing was completely out of the
hands of the physicians. The requirements were controlled by the
state legislatures, and at the time the lawmakers were in the process
of repealing the medical license laws, making it possible for anyone
who claimed to be a physician to open an office and practice
medicine. The question of whether the colleges or the societies
should license physicians was solved, then, by the solons who
decided that physicians did not have to be licensed.

Now that the organization that soon became known as the American Medical Association had investigated the need for reform and
adopted two resolutions, state and local societies began discussing
the ways to enforce the decisions made at the convention. Typical
were the debates that took place in Cincinnati at meetings of the
Hamilton County Medical Club. On July 18, 1847, Professor John P.
Harrison of the Medical College of Ohio defended the medical
schools against the continuing attacks by leading physicians. He
declared that in spite of what some had said, medical education was

not all that bad. He compared it with conditions thirty years earlier when there were few schools and fewer branches of medical science. Back in 1814, he said, "Cullen was read by a few, but Old Thomas was the favorite author, and constituted the whole library of many." "In moral dignity, and purity," there was a great improvement. "In '14," he declared, "almost all prominent medical men of the West were avowed Infidels; and very large numbers [were] addicted to habits of intemperance."[7]

Other physicians in attendance disagreed with much of what Harrison had said. They argued that the American physicians were clearly inferior to those in Europe, and they defended the morality of the previous generation. Dr. Lakey insisted that in 1814 the physicians "along the Atlantic Coast were not generally infidels," and as proof he mentioned "the name and influence" of Benjamin Rush. Dr. Robert Thompson of Columbus slightly changed the subject when he agreed with Dr. Bartles who had said at the 1846 AMA convention that the great problem was that the medical professors conferred degrees and licenses on poorly trained men. Thompson argued for the establishment of a state medical society with the power to supervise medical education and examine all applicants for both degrees and licenses. Harrison rushed to the defense of his colleagues on the faculty, arguing vehemently against the separation of teaching from awarding degrees.[8]

On August 4, 1847, Dr. Lakey read a paper on medical education before the Hamilton County Medical Club. He described the work of the AMA at its Philadelphia convention, emphasizing the proposed standards of preliminary education. At that convention, it was argued that students should have a good English education as well as a knowledge of natural philosophy, math, Latin, and Greek. Lakey said that everyone agreed on the need for students to have a good English education, but he disagreed with the rest of the requirements. Chemistry and medical botany, he said, were all that was needed of natural philosophy, and he thought that mathematics, Greek, and Latin were totally unnecessary for physicians.[9]

Although Lakey did not accept the AMA proposal on preliminary education, he admitted that the medical profession had retrograded in the past forty years. "The people had grown more intelligent; but the profession had not improved in a similar ratio." He advocated

that the colleges revive the bachelor's degree and refrain from conferring the doctorate on men less than forty years of age. In addition,
Lakey insisted on an impartial board examining all applicants to the
colleges in order to ensure that only qualified students would be
admitted and ultimately graduated as physicians. Once again, Harrison rushed to defend the faculty. He said that the preceptors should
accept only those students who could demonstrate a good preliminary education, but he insisted that the colleges had an obligation to
admit "such students however ignorant as the preceptors chose to
send them."[10]

Alvah H. Baker, a founder of the Cincinnati College of Medicine
and Surgery, once a "great stickler for a preliminary education," told
his colleagues that he had changed his mind when he learned that
both Daniel Drake and John Eberle, the medical writer, had limited
backgrounds. Baker agreed with Harrison that the colleges should
admit anyone who chose to study medicine. He sarcastically noted
that education had hurt many people, most notably the clergymen
who patronized and endorsed the "steamers, eclectics and other
quacks."

The problem facing medical education was obvious; the two physicians with college affiliations insisted that the schools had to admit
everyone who chose to attend, regardless of their previous education. Another participant, Dr. Lace, agreed that the schools had to
admit all students sent by preceptors, but he noted that the colleges
did not have to graduate all their students. "The Schools," he said,
had "in a great measure lost sight of the higher objects for which they
were instituted." Instead, they seemed "to have entered upon an
ignoble rivalship to see which could have the greatest number of
students."[11]

The subject of preliminary education provoked the most debate.
The advocates of classical training argued that the best way to ensure
graduation of well-qualified physicians was to require all students to
have a good English education as well as a knowledge of natural
philosophy, mathematics, Latin, and Greek. In that way, illiterates
would no longer become medical students or physicians. The opponents of classical education argued, also quite correctly, that students
in the West and South had little opportunity to acquire the necessary
classical training. Indeed, even on the East Coast, only sons of

wealthy families could afford what the AMA had proposed as standards of preliminary education. Sons of the middle classes attended the common schools, which did not teach Latin and Greek.[12]

In 1847, J. K. Mitchell of the Jefferson Medical College declared that a student from "the wild and remote part of our country" had no choice but to be totally ignorant of Latin and Greek. The colleges could not discriminate, he said, against a student who happened to be raised in an area with no schools. If he wanted to become a physician, the medical colleges provided the opportunity for someone "with laudable zeal," who "emerges from the grand old woods, or leaps from the boundless prairie." Mitchell said that in any case, it was possible to acquire the necessary preliminary education during the college recess![13]

On the other hand, Samuel Jackson of the University of Pennsylvania, in making the annual discourse before the Philadelphia County Medical Society, declared that high standards would not deter the "superior man" who enters the profession. In spite of the overwhelming odds, the determined boy would acquire the education. "As Hannibal broke down the Alps . . . and opened his way to the regions of sunshine," Jackson rhetorically exclaimed, "so will this fiery boy open his way to the profession of medicine."[14]

In May 1847 when the Ohio Medical Convention gathered, the delegates had a lengthy discussion on ways to improve medical education. Finally a motion was adopted requesting the professors in Ohio's medical colleges to report on the measures, "if any, they have taken to carry out the recommendations" made by the AMA.[15] When they reconvened in May 1848, the medical professors were ready with their reports. J. P. Kirtland described the program at the Cleveland Medical College, John S. Butterfield described the situation at the Starling Medical College, and Reuben D. Mussey, who had attended the 1827 Northampton convention as a delegate from Dartmouth, informed them of the requirements at the Medical College of Ohio. It was obvious that the colleges had made no attempt to comply with the recommendations of the AMA.

Dr. David Judkins next offered a resolution stating that whereas the representatives of the colleges "have informed this Convention that the institutions with which they are connected, have taken no steps whatever to advance the cause of Medical Education . . . and yet they all agree that there are crying evils in this respect . . . this convention urges, upon the Professors . . . the necessity of uniting" to carry out the AMA plan for reforming medical education. After a great deal of debate and several parliamentary maneuvers, the physicians adopted a substitute resolution, which did not explicitly condemn the professors.[16]

As time passed, it became more and more obvious that the colleges were not about to make changes in their requirements, especially at a time when anyone could practice medicine without having attended medical college. The professors were realistic in their fears that a reform of medical education might destroy the lifeblood of the college, the ever-increasing stream of unqualified students sent by the preceptors.

When the American Medical Association met in Baltimore on May 2, 1848, there had been little change. The hopes and dreams of the reformers had gone unanswered. Nathaniel Chapman said in his presidential address that the medical profession had faced "difficulties and dangers, arising mainly from the too ready admixture into it of individuals unworthy of the association, either by intellectual culture, or moral discipline, by whom it is abased."[17]

The AMA committee on medical education presented a report that reiterated the earlier statements on preliminary education and graduation requirements. The committee emphasized the need for clinical instruction and recommended that hospitals open their wards to teaching and that the schools "resort to every honorable means to obtain access for their students to the Wards of well-regulated hospitals." The committee proposed that medical students be examined in the presence of the profession at large to prevent the graduation of incompetents.[18] Of course, since the association had no way of enforcing its recommendations and since the colleges were not about to make any reforms, the AMA was merely a moral force, which at the time seemed little better than no force at all.

Committees of the AMA investigated the existing conditions in the profession, which added to the drive for medical reform. Circulars were sent to all the county clerks in Virginia, asking for information on the physicians who were actively practicing medicine. Two-thirds of the clerks responded. The returns indicated that 678 of the 972 physicians in those counties had received degrees from medical colleges. More than one-quarter of the physicians, 249, practiced medicine without any authority at all; 228 of those had not devoted even one hour to medical study. A large proportion of these latter "physicians" practiced in the western counties of the state.[19]

A similar survey of physicians in Delaware indicated that 28 percent of the physicians in the state were not medical graduates. In addition, 21 percent of the practicing physicians were neither graduates nor licensed to practice medicine.[20] These statistics indicated clearly that a high percentage of the so-called physicians were totally unqualified, being neither medical graduates nor licensed (or registered) to practice medicine.

The need for reform was obvious, but the AMA committee on medical education could do little more than "remind" the colleges of the 1847 resolutions on preliminary education and graduation requirements. In 1849 the committee recommended that six months of hospital instruction be required for graduation and then proposed that state medical societies be established where none existed as the first step to medical reform.[21]

Rather significantly, American medical reform was once again influenced by the European example. By the 1830s, as a result of the establishment of large teaching hospitals and the influence of Pierre Louis, Paris had replaced Edinburgh as the mecca of the American physician. An analysis of the records indicates that 222 American doctors visited Paris in the 1830s, and at least sixty-seven of them taught in American medical schools either before or after their European experience. For instance, five members of the Harvard medical faculty had studied in Paris: J. C. Warren, Henry I. Bowditch, Henry J. Bigelow, J. B. S. Jackson, and George Shattuck, Jr. Of course, it was difficult for one college to reform without driving students to other institutions, but because so many leading physicians had seen the superiority of French clinical methods, with its extensive use of hospitals in medical education, the stage was set for a widespread drive to initiate French methods in the American colleges. In fact, many of those who were active in the American Medical Association committee on medical education had been educated in Paris. In 1849 the committee recommended the French emphasis on clinical teaching and dissection.[22]

The committee submitted an elaborate 120-page study of American medical education, comparing it to conditions in Europe and examining the legal requirements in each state. The study indicated that twenty-two of the thirty-eight colleges had seven or more professors; that four schools had increased their term to six months or more; that ten schools still did not require a certificate from preceptors; that only seventeen schools required dissection; and that only in seven was hospital attendance required. [23]

Interestingly, two years after the AMA had insisted on lengthening the course to six months, the Harvard medical faculty presented a defense of the four-month course of lectures. The Harvard faculty, represented by Jacob Bigelow, Oliver Wendell Holmes, and John Ware, argued that lecturing was an inadequate way of imparting or gaining knowledge; lengthening the lecture term, they said, would not ensure the graduation of better physicians. The faculty suggested that private study take up the remaining eight months of the year; only through work with preceptors and study in hospitals could the students acquire the knowledge and experience necessary for successful practice. [24]

Although the logic of the Harvard professors was flawless, Harvard was typical of the American colleges of the day: it made no changes in response to the AMA standards. In 1849, Harvard still had a four-month course of lectures and did not require dissection. In addition, increasing the time of formal medical study by 50 percent, from eight months to twelve months, could not possibly have had a detrimental effect on the students. In any case, the AMA established a committee, consisting of Samuel Jackson, John L. Atlee, and Alfred Stillé, to prepare a statement defending the six-month course of study. [25]

Actually, two schools did make changes in their programs to conform to the recommended AMA standards. In 1847 the University of Pennsylvania and New York's College of Physicians and Surgeons advertised their newly developed six-month course of lectures. The result was disaster. The Jefferson Medical College continued its four-month course, and as a result, its class "increased more rapidly than it had ever before," until its enrollment "far outnumbered that of the University." Within six years, the University of Pennsylvania was forced to abandon its well-intentioned experiment. [26]

The editor of *The Stethoscope,* a journal published in Richmond, sadly noted that two courageous colleges could not effect a reformation. This was especially true "when thirty-odd other medical colleges were resisting these reforms, and underbidding in the standards of requirement for the doctorate." The editor was particularly upset that the opponents of medical reform were arguing that the failure of reform at those two schools was evidence that the medical schools had to maintain low standards or go out of business. He likened the situation to the military. "If the commander of an army orders his forces to storm a fortification," he said, "and all but two regiments should retreat in an opposite direction," the latter cannot point "to the mangled corpses of those who had gloriously fallen in discharge of duty, as proof that the orders of the commander were unwise."[27]

In 1851 one of the most active supporters of medical reform, Yale's Worthington Hooker, read the report of the AMA committee on medical education. He reminded the faculties of the 1847 standards of medical education and declared that the abuses "demand the serious consideration of the profession." He said that the "free discussion" of the abuses was "an important means of effecting their removal," but he argued that due to the political realities of the day, public opinion must be reformed before any medical reform could ever succeed. Hooker described how most students were educated. For eight months they "read" medicine in some physician's office. For the next four months they heard from four to seven lectures daily, attended hospital clinics, if that was required, and practiced dissection "if they incline to do so." There was no graduation in the curriculum—no preparation in terms of studying one course as prerequisite for a more difficult one. Hooker concluded that "all is acquired in a very loose and confused manner." After two years, the student was graduated, even though he may never have seen a patient, he may never have learned anatomy by dissection, and he may have been totally unprepared to practice medicine.[28]

By 1854 and 1855, it seemed apparent that the AMA had failed to bring about the needed reform in medical education. David M. Reese, the editor of the *American Medical Gazette*, wrote in 1855: "The conviction appears to be general, among writers" that the association had been wholly unsuccessful. He said that "notwithstanding the numerous reforms attempted, recommended and resolved on by repeated *'whereases'* and reiterated at every successive

meeting, by high-sounding resolutions, and published in each
volume of the *Transactions,* yet in *effectuating any one of these,
after seven years' trial, the efforts of the Association in this regard
have resulted in signal and utter failure."* [29]

Even Thomas Blachford, a Troy, New York, physician and a firm
advocate of medical reform, had to come to the same conclusion. He
noted that "the doctors come together . . . in grand consultation,
once a year. They feel the pulse, notice the tongue, examine the
intellectual secretions" and "agree upon a prescription. . . . But
either the pill prepared has been too big for the throat, or the throat
too constricted for the pill." He believed the basic problem was that
unless the government granted to the AMA the power to license
physicians and confer degrees, "it seems futile" to do more than ask
voluntary compliance, unless the AMA is willing to make compliance
a "test of membership." Blachford thought, however, that such a
radical course of action would "be to cut off at one swoop nearly all
our colleges," and it would "seem almost like a death blow" to the
association. [30]

By the time of the 1857 Nashville convention, the AMA members
and delegates were becoming frustrated at their inability to bring
about the reforms in medical education that would raise the prestige
and influence of the entire profession. In the midst of this disappointment, Jesse Boring of Georgia resolved "that this Assocation has not
the power to control the subject of medical education" and that any
further attempt to do so "would not only be useless, but calculated to
disturb and distract the deliberations of this Association."[31]

After some debate, R. C. Currey of Tennessee offered a substitute
establishing a five-man committee "who are in no way connected
with any Medical School" and directing it to develop a system of
medical instruction and to submit a report in 1858. Currey's motion
also stated that after the recommendations were adopted, those
colleges that accepted them would be represented at AMA conventions, while the others would forever be ostracized from the
"respectable" branch of the profession. A committee was established
consisting of George R. Grant of Memphis, René La Roche of
Philadelphia, C. B. Nottingham of Macon, Georgia, John Watson of
New York City, and James R. Wood of New York City. [32]

Although this action might have destroyed the American Medical

Association, as Blachford suggested, the delegates apparently considered it a necessary step. Indeed, the AMA had been established back in 1846 in order to reform medical education and raise the prestige of the entire profession. Since the colleges had ignored all requests for "voluntary compliance" with the increased standards, either the AMA could be disbanded as a total failure or it could take a moral stance by demanding compliance as a test of membership. The members of the AMA considered themselves defenders of professional morality; they believed they could cast aside any colleges that refused to comply, considering them "irregular" institutions. The choice was clear for the AMA: it could either admit defeat or it could fight to force colleges to comply with the accepted standards of medical education. By adopting Currey's motion, the AMA chose to fight.

When the association reconvened in Washington, D.C., in 1858, the committee reported that the best way to bring about reform was for the colleges to hold their own convention just before the next AMA meeting. The colleges would devise a uniform system of education and report back to the AMA.[33] This was an intelligent decision. Because the colleges would only establish standards they could accept, letting the colleges devise their own standards guaranteed that a number of them would fully adhere to the "AMA" standards of medical education. If the delegates to the AMA convention had developed their own standards, they might have discovered that not one college would accept them.

Representatives of twenty-one colleges gathered in Louisville at the appointed time in 1859, the day before the AMA meeting. They represented about half the schools in a disappointing geographical distribution. All the delegates were from western and southern institutions, except for professors from Dartmouth, Harvard, and the Jefferson Medical College. In order to expedite business a five-man committee was directed to make specific proposals, and it was given thirty minutes to do so.[34]

The committee, which included N. S. Davis, Moses Gunn of the University of Michigan, H. R. Frost of the Medical College of South Carolina, George C. Shattuck of Harvard, and Lunsford P. Yandell of the University of Louisville, proposed a number of resolutions. First, they agreed that the AMA standards should be rigidly enforced. They urged the AMA to adopt measures to enforce its standards of preliminary education. Second, the committee recommended that no college be allowed to substitute medical practice for a course of lectures. This was a response to the fact that some institutions gave advanced standing to men who had practiced medicine without having attended any college. Third, the committee declared that clinical instruction constituted a necessary part of medical education and that every degree candidate should be required to devote at least five months to clinical work. Finally, it proposed that every college enforce the rule requiring three full years of medical study before graduation and that a diploma from any college violating this rule should not be recognized as valid.[35]

After a lengthy debate, it was decided that since so many schools were not represented, no changes should be made unless generally accepted. Therefore, by a vote of ten to nine, the delegates decided to adjourn to the day before the next AMA convention after appointing a committee to confer with the various schools and to make further recommendations. The committee included G. C. Blackman of the Medical College of Ohio, H. F. Campbell of the Medical College of Georgia, Moses Gunn of the University of Michigan, George C. Shattuck of Harvard, and L. P. Yandell of the University of Louisville. Dixi Crosby of Dartmouth reported the decisions to the AMA, and he suggested that a similar committee be appointed to confer with the teachers' committee. The "lay" committee was duly organized, including Thomas Blachford, Nathan Bozeman of Montgomery, Alabama, William Brodie of Detroit, D. Francis Condie of Philadelphia, and W. C. Sneed of Frankfort, Kentucky.[36]

The two committees corresponded with each other and met three times prior to the 1860 New Haven convention. In a series of proposals to the AMA they recommended that the colleges require a certificate of three years' study with a regularly educated preceptor and evidence of having taken two full courses of lectures in two separate years. The committee recommended that the AMA not recognize as regularly organized any college that did not require evidence of a suitable preliminary education. In addition, every student should be required to devote four months to clinical study in a hospital. Two or three delegates of the state medical societies should be present and voting at the examination of all degree candidates. Further, the committee recommended that the colleges and the professorships be endowed so they would not be as dependent on the students for their income. Finally, they suggested that the AMA not allow representation to any college that did not comply with these rules. The AMA convention adopted the entire package.[37]

Unfortunately for the cause of medical reform, the Civil War was just over the horizon. When Lincoln's election led to secession and ultimately to war, the events of the day completely overshadowed the problems of the colleges. A great many physicians, North and South, dedicated their next few years either to the cause of the Union or states' rights, and the actions of the AMA were soon forgotten. All of this occurred at precisely the time when the AMA had determined to take its stand in the battle to reform medical education; it had to wait to complete its struggle, for the survival of the nation was at stake on a larger battleground.

Notes

1. *Proceedings of the National Medical Conventions Held in New York, May, 1846, and in Philadelphia, May, 1847* (Philadelphia, 1847), pp. 63-68.

2. Ibid., p. 70.

3. Ibid., pp. 73-74.

4. Ibid., pp. 79-82.

5. Ibid., pp. 115-123.

6. Ibid., pp. 107-113. Cock supported both the majority and minority reports.

7. Hamilton County Medical Club, minutes, July 18, 1847, National Library of Medicine, Bethesda, Maryland.

8. Ibid.

9. Ibid., August 4, 1847.

10. Ibid.

11. Ibid.

12. For a defense of the low standards on economic and class grounds, see *Nashville Journal of Medicine and Science* 19 (October 1860): 327-330.

13. J. K. Mitchell, *Lecture Introductory to the Course on the Practice of Medicine in the Jefferson Medical College* (Philadelphia, 1847), pp. 15-16. See also Robert M. Huston, *Lecture Introductory to the Course on Materia Medica and General Therapeutics* (Philadelphia, 1852), pp. 11-17.

14. Samuel Jackson, *Medical Education* (Philadelphia, 1853), p. 10. For an argument in favor of a good English education, see Thomas D. Mitchell, *The Study of Medicine* (Philadelphia, 1849), esp. pp. 16-17.

15. *Proceedings of the Ohio Medical Convention* (Columbus, 1847), pp. 10-11.

16. *Proceedings of the Ohio Medical Convention* (Columbus, 1848), pp. 6-7.

17. *Transactions of the American Medical Association* 1 (1848): 8.

18. Ibid., 235-247.

19. Ibid., 359-364.

20. Ibid., 365ff.

21. Ibid. 2 (1849): 40-41.

22. Russell M. Jones, "American Doctors and the Parisian Medical World, 1830-1840," *Bulletin of the History of Medicine* 47 (January-February 1973): 40-65; (March-April 1973): 177-204. See also Walter R. Steiner, "Some Distinguished American Medical Students of Pierre-Charles-Alexander Louis of Paris," *Bulletin of the History of Medicine* 7 (1939): 783-793.

23. *Transactions of the AMA* 2 (1849): 281-299.

24. Ibid., 353-358.

25. Ibid., 43-44, 284-285, 359-370.

26. *St. Louis Medical and Surgical Journal* 12 (August 1854): 471. See also William Pepper, *Higher Medical Education* (Philadelphia, 1894), pp. 24-25.

27. *The Stethoscope* 4 (November 1854): 647.

28. *Transactions of the AMA* 4 (1851): 34-35, 409-446.

29. Quoted in Morris Fishbein, *History of the American Medical Association* (Philadelphia and London, 1947), p. 65.

30. Thomas Blachford, "A Condensed Statement of What Has Been Attempted for the Advancement of Medical Education, by the Medical Conventions of 1846 and 1847, and by the A.M.A. Since Its Organization in 1847," in *Transactions, Medical Society of the State of New York, 1860* (Albany, 1860), pp. 136-137.

31. *Transactions of the AMA* 10 (1857): 27-29.

32. Ibid.

33. Ibid. 11 (1858): 31-35.

34. *Atlanta Medical Journal* 4 (June 1859): 640-642. See also Blachford, "A Condensed Statement," pp. 120-138.

35. Ibid.

36. Ibid.

37. *Transactions of the AMA* 13 (1860): 31-35.

7

The Situation Deteriorates Further, 1860-1890

With the end of the war, physicians once again turned their attention to medical education. In 1866 the American Medical Association resumed its drive to reform American medical education, this time in concert with a number of the colleges. Delegates of some western schools had agreed to extend their terms to six months, "provided that the other colleges . . . did the same." When this was reported to the AMA, N. S. Davis moved that the association "request the medical colleges to hold a convention for thoroughly revising the whole system of medical college instruction." This was unanimously adopted, and a five-man committee, consisting of Davis, Worthington Hooker, George C. Shattuck, Samuel D. Gross of the Jefferson Medical College, and M. B. Wright of the Medical College of Ohio, was established to make all the necessary arrangements.[1]

The convention of teachers was held on May 3, 1867, the day before the AMA was to convene in Cincinnati. Only nineteen colleges sent delegates, but by now a disappointing turnout was expected by those interested in medical reform. The professors elected Alfred Stillé of the University of Pennslyvania as chairman, and then they got down to work. After some debate, a series of resolutions was approved, which represented the most far-reaching proposals for reform that had ever been made by such a committee. It was agreed that there should be a "positive standard" of preliminary education and that every student should be required to either undergo an examination or present evidence of a good educational foundation. The teachers agreed that no college should have a term of less than six months and that the students be required to study for four years, including three courses of lectures.

The convention decided that no college should have fewer than nine professors and that there should be a graded curriculum to systematize medical study. According to the proposal, the first year would be devoted to courses in descriptive anatomy through dissection, physiology and histology, inorganic chemistry, materia medica, and therapeutics; in the second year the students would learn organic chemistry, toxicology, pathology, morbid anatomy, surgical anatomy, and surgery, as well as public hygiene, medical jurisprudence, and medical ethics. The third year would provide practical work in medicine, surgery, obstetrics, and diseases of women and children, and there would be clinical work in local hospitals. In order to advance to the next year of studies, students would be required to pass examinations on the courses taken in each year.

The teachers voted that the colleges must develop "some effectual methods of ascertaining the actual attendance of students," rather than simply assuming that possession of a lecture ticket was evidence of proficiency. Finally, a committee was appointed to present the resolutions to the faculties of the colleges, "with a view to the early and simultaneous practical adoption."[2]

The AMA endorsed the plan, and a committee prepared a statement in support of the proposition. The report declared that the reform would "erect an effectual barrier against the disgraceful practice of conferring the distinguished title of Doctor of Medicine upon men so illiterate that they cannot write an ordinary business letter in creditable English." It would transform medical education from a hodgepodge of lectures into a systematic course of studies, with the fundamental branches "preparatory to the practical." Most important, the reforms "would neither alter the relative position of the several colleges to each other, nor diminish the aggregate number of students annually attending, nor materially increase the annual expenditure of any," as long as all the colleges accepted the proposals. The increased number of professors would "be more than compensated for by requiring all students to attend and pay for three annual courses instead of two." Finally, the AMA committee noted that the reforms did not require any aid from the legislatures; all that was needed was the cooperation of the colleges.[3]

By the next year, N. S. Davis was able to report that "evident progress was being made" in the proposals to reform medical education. "Several schools," he said, "had indorsed the plan."[4] After the delegates to the AMA convention heard his report, they supported a motion that the whole subject of medical education be referred to the faculties of the colleges, with the association "pledging itself to adopt and enforce any system or plan that may be agreed upon by two-thirds of all recognized medical colleges."[5] By adopting this motion, the AMA in effect had washed its hands of medical education, once again leaving it up to the colleges. It was a step in the wrong direction; more than two-thirds of the schools had low standards and had shown little inclination to make any reforms.

When the AMA convened in New Orleans in 1869, the meeting began on a sour note. In his presidential address William O. Baldwin painted a dismal picture of American medical education. "Any man can enter a medical college in this country," he exclaimed, "without having gone through even the jest or mockery of spending a year in a private preceptor's office." Anyone was admitted to the colleges "by simply paying the fees required." Those who so desired would attend the lectures and hold private quiz-clubs to familiarize themselves with the material, while many of the other students attended the "lager-beer saloons and theatres at night." Standards were so low, the president declared, that it was "but a short step from the plough-handles to the diploma."[6] Baldwin wanted the colleges to unite and establish some "uniform and elevated standards of requirements," but he felt that it was "almost a Utopian idea, a forlorn hope." This path to reform, he said, must be abandoned. There was no hope for reform, he exclaimed, "except through FEDERAL LEGISLATION."[7]

The committee on medical education made its report, which demonstrated how foolish it was to expect reform to come from *any* legislature. The committee, which included J. C. Reeve of Ohio and

W. C. McCook of Pennsylvania, described the process of reform in Ohio. In the 1866-1867 legislative session a bill was introduced to regulate the practice of medicine by requiring all graduates to be examined by a committee of the state medical society. The proposal included several safeguards to minimize opposition: it would not interfere with those already practicing, regardless of their competence, and there would be no examination in materia medica and therapeutics, to allay the fears of the unorthodox practitioners. Yet the bill failed to pass, and the orthodox profession did not "heartily and unitedly" support it. The next measure introduced would have made it illegal to practice without a diploma from some medical college. Because Ohio had already chartered a homeopathic, an eclectic, and a "physio-vital" college, it was believed that all the physicians could unite in support of a bill that would prevent practice by men who were totally uneducated. This bill was passed by the legislature, but with an amendment making a certificate from any county society a license to practice medicine. As some county societies had low standards, this was a gaping loophole.

After reviewing the situation in Ohio, the AMA committee concluded that legislative aid was not forthcoming and that the only possible way to solve the problems of medical education was for the AMA to set standards and enforce them by condemning schools that did not abide by the reforms and considering their graduates as irregular practitioners.[8] Presumably, no self-respecting member of a county and state medical society would send students to an unaccredited college, which meant that the enrollment of any college in that category would decrease.

After Baldwin's presidential address and the report of the committee on medical education, N. S. Davis declared that the past twenty-five years of the drive to reform medical education had been a dismal failure. Because the colleges would not reform themselves, Davis agreed with the proposals of the committee on medical education. He moved that each state society appoint boards to examine all who wanted to practice medicine and that the examining boards insist on "proper general education" of all applicants. The motion further stated that when two-thirds of the societies had established such a system, the AMA would deny representation to members of the other societies and treat them as irregular practitioners. Davis hoped that the value of a diploma could be reduced by forcing the colleges "to rival each other in the extent and efficiency of their course of instruction, instead of the number of diplomas which they can annually distribute." The AMA adopted this plan, and it empowered a committee to carry it out. The committee included Davis, Joseph M. Toner (the medical biographer), and Job S. Weatherly of Alabama.[9]

In 1871 the committee sadly reported that very little progress had been made. The state medical societies of Kansas, Maryland, New Jersey, and Wisconsin had approved the proposals; the societies of New York and New Hampshire had tabled consideration of the motion; the societies in Alabama, Illinois, Indiana, Iowa, Kentucky, Michigan, Ohio, and Pennsylvania had referred the matter to committees that had not yet replied; the other state societies had taken no action whatever.[10] The 1869 attempt to reform medical education had been a failure.

In 1870 a convention of medical teachers once again gathered prior to the AMA convention. Nineteen schools sent delegates, which once again represented a minority of the total number (about sixty) of colleges. There were no representatives from the New York City or Boston colleges. The professors began by discussing the proposals that had been made at the last meeting of the group in 1867.

During the debate, Alfred Stillé moved that the propositions were praiseworthy and "if they could be generally carried into effect, [they] would tend to elevate the medical profession." Requirements, he said, "must be practically determined by each Medical College by itself, by the average attainments of its students, and by other considerations of which it alone can judge." Stillé's motion requested the colleges to try to conform to the earlier plan, but left it up to the individual colleges. His motion was defeated "by a decided majority." Considering his earlier insistence on stringent regulations, one can only assume that Stillé had been directed by his faculty to present that motion. At that point, Professors J. B. Johnson of the St. Louis Medical College and Samuel Bemiss of the University of Louisiana asked how many delegates were empowered to bind their schools to the decisions of the convention. Only two of the professors could do that—Johnson and Bemiss. N. S. Davis of the Chicago Medical College and Samuel Logan of the New Orleans School of Medicine said that they could pledge to any "reasonable measures of reform."

The other delegates did not really represent their colleges. This meant that the deliberations at the convention were just so many words; this realization destroyed any hope that the gathering might effect a real change. At that recognition, Stillé's motion was reconsidered and adopted.[11]

Bemiss reported his impressions to the faculty of the University of Louisiana. He sadly exclaimed that "there is not at this time, nor at any discernible period in the future, the slightest hope of any general cooperation" of medical schools. The attempt at united action, he said, was "miserable and humiliating." Since united action was hopeless, individual action "was even more so" because any improvement in standards at one school would decrease enrollment. The university had considered the need for reform, but Bemiss rejected it as self-defeating. After all, he said, reform at any school would strengthen "the less worthy colleges" by driving students elsewhere in search of "a quick diploma."[12]

The medical faculty of the University of Louisiana (which later became the Tulane Medical School) included a number of advocates of reform. One of these was Stanford Chaillé, professor of physiology and anatomy. In a brilliant analysis of the problems of medical education, Chaillé examined every possible avenue of reform. State laws establishing examining boards would be an ideal solution, he said. That would eliminate the detrimental influence of the students, because colleges no longer could lower requirements, if students had to pass examinations administered by outsiders in order to practice medicine. Chaillé recognized that Americans were jealous of restrictive laws and would "not submit to limitations of that personal freedom." There could be no reform until the people became convinced that "freedom lost will be more than compensated for by the benefits gained." Chaillé was especially dubious about the future of reform in Louisiana. He noted that "conservative Louisiana" had repealed the old medical license laws, and so, he asked, "What can any good citizen hope from radical Africanized" Louisiana? If the best-governed northern states had "utterly failed to reform medical education," he said, "what can the misgoverned Southern States hope to accomplish?"[13]

Chaillé concluded that there was no hope for reform until public opinion became enlightened enough to recognize the need for improving the quality of medical care. The role of the profession, therefore, was to advance science and educate the public in the laws of "health, life, and nature." A first step, he said, could be to eradicate smallpox, which in 1873 alone killed more than five hundred people in New Orleans. He predicted that when the people realized the importance of public health, public opinion would gradually shift and the citizenry would be able to "estimate and secure the best measures and men to guard their health."[14]

Over the years, several individuals had proposed that it might be possible to initiate reform by establishing a national medical college with the highest standards. Presumably it would set an example for the other schools by producing superior practitioners. As a result, the other colleges would be so obviously inferior that they would be forced to emulate the national institution.[15] At the 1871 AMA convention, Francis G. Smith of the University of Pennsylvania, chairman of a committee established to investigate the possibility of such a plan, reported that a national medical school was not feasible at present, "in consequence of the political antagonisms, complications, and tendencies of the country." A bill for such a school had been introduced in Congress, but irregular practitioners were demanding that they be allowed to participate; the last thing the AMA wanted was to establish a national medical school that recognized and taught homeopathy. The committee concluded: "To trust to politicians for the advancement of scientific medicine would be to seek . . . such protection as wolves give to lambs." Moreover, since politicians were unable "to judge of medical qualifications," there would be "so many selfish interests at work that the selection of suitable professors could probably never be made." The committee concluded, however, that it "cannot believe . . . that this great country will *always* be behind the civilization of the world" and that action might be more appropriate at some time in the future.[16]

At the same convention Eli Geddings, who had taught medicine for more than fifty years in South Carolina, presented his report on medical education. He complained about the proliferation of the colleges. The politicians "have showered them upon us like the locusts from the desert, and," he said, "like those myrmidons of destruction, they have blighted and defiled, wherever most numerous, all the beauty, and verdure, and freshness of the fair domain of medical science." "Under the present state of legislation," he continued, "every town and village bids fair to become the seat of a temple of Aesculapius," or of Thomson, Hahnemann, Priesnitz, Mesmer, Baunscheidt, and other unorthodox practitioners who had followers enough to establish medical sects.[17] Geddings concluded that as long as "medical teaching, and its associated 'diploma traffic,' are allowed to remain without check or restraint in the hands of a number of 'stock-jobbing' corporations called Medical Colleges," the abuses would remain. He predicted that it would ultimately result "in the utter downfall of scientific medicine in the United States, and the inauguration of a universal system of Quackery."[18]

Dr. Henry D. Holton of Vermont moved that each state and local society provide a board of censors to determine the educational qualifications of the students, and that until a student could present a certificate from the censor or a degree from a literary college of good standing, no member of any society would be permitted to allow him in his office. This motion was adopted, and the same committee that had been established to oversee a similar proposal in 1869 was reappointed—Davis, Toner, and Weatherly.[19]

Not much came of these attempts by the AMA to bring about reform in medical education. The association simply was not strong enough to enforce its decisions. Indeed when the AMA adopted a resolution declaring that it had the power to set standards of education and that it would consider colleges which did not reform as irregular institutions, the association was bitterly condemned by no less than Henry J. Bigelow, the Harvard professor. In June 1871 Bigelow read a paper before the Massachusetts Medical Society, "Medical Education in America," in which he denounced the AMA's attempts to control medical education. The delegates to the national conventions, he said, "pronounce immature opinions, claim for themselves authority, and hastily denounce friends." They even went so far, Bigelow noted, as issuing "bulls of excommunication," which were, he said, of "as little significance as the tail of a comet, which may overcast the whole country with its shadow, but which astronomers assure us may be carried in a man's hat." The Harvard professor concluded by declaring unequivocally: "A body of so uncertain temper and impulsive action obviously has no authority to express even public medical Opinion."[20]

The AMA was trying to find some solution to the problem of medical education, but to no avail. A number of dedicated men worked long and hard to effect the reformation, men who included N. S. Davis, Worthington Hooker, and Joseph Toner, but very few colleges were willing to increase standards when that almost certainly would have meant losing a large number of students to schools that refused to reform.

The situation was becoming even more scandalous. The colleges were not reforming to any significant extent, and the medical profession still did not attract the best students. Charles McIntyre made a study of the percentage of college graduates who went on to become physicians, and he demonstrated that relatively few graduates entered the profession. From 1801 to 1825, 10.4 percent of all college graduates eventually became physicians. Since 1825, the percentage had fallen to 9.2, as compared to 21 percent who studied theology and 19.7 percent who went into law. McIntyre concluded that it was a "mistake" to classify "the *medical business* among the learned professions."[21]

In an address before the New Hampshire State Medical Society, Lyman B. How described the case of a typical student, "Sam Bucus." Bucus "never intended to be anything but a farmer" until his father became ill. The physician who was called "put a little morphine on his tongue" and charged $1.25. Sam was impressed by the easy way to earn money; he decided to become a physician. Bucus applied to "Dr. Physic," who "was pleased with the idea of having a student," especially one who would "be so useful about taking care of his office and horse, . . . and trying to collect his bills."

Sam became a medical student, and he devoted his time to "reading" medicine. He had "the free range of the doctor's library of ten volumes." After a year and a half of study, he went to college. But because his preliminary education had been so limited, he did poorly in medical school; for example, he handed in a "poorly written, misspelled and unpunctuated thesis on typhoid fever." But he did have some redeeming attributes. He had "an excellent character, a desire to do about right, a possibility that he will not hurt anybody," and he had "fifteen or twenty dollars for a diploma." He graduated, returned home, and began to practice medicine.[22]

In 1881, William W. Green, the president of the Maine Medical

Association, said that the greatest defect in medical education was the system of preceptorship. Green made the point that any physician could have students, and every certificate of three years' study was accepted by the colleges. "Just think of it!" he declared. "No matter whether he has a library, dissecting-rooms, chemical laboratory, microscope or not . . . if he has a diploma, and occupies a nominal position in the profession, he is competent, under the law, to take charge and direction" of medical education.[23]

The inevitable result was the admission to the profession of "a large class of men" who were "utterly unfit for the work as regards preliminary education." Yet physicians were "anxious" to attract students. Green noted that there was "a certain *eclat* attached to preceptorship," as well as convenience for the physician. In addition, too many physicians sympathized with men "who, having failed in other pursuits, look to the practice of medicine as a *dernier ressort* for retrieving broken fortunes."[24]

Finally, Green complained, a great many apprentices never spent any time with their preceptors. Only those who could afford to devote their time to the study of medicine would stay in the doctor's office. A few would work for the physician, paying for room and board with their labor. Most students, however, were not wealthy. They had to teach school or work on farms, in mills, or elsewhere; these men read medicine in their spare time, only occasionally calling on the preceptor.[25]

In his autobiography, Isaac Abt, the prominent pediatrician, described the students at the Chicago Medical College when he enrolled in the 1870s. He noted that the entrance requirements "did not bar many who were insufficiently prepared." A few of the students were college graduates, most were from high schools, and some had received their only preparation in elementary school. "They came from shops and factories, farms and mines; one had been a preacher, one a barber, another an iceman."[26]

It was ludicrous for such unprepared students to attend medical school. The professors were reported to have "wasted" their time trying "to teach anatomy, to demonstrate the cochlea, the lamina spirilis, scala vestibuli and scala tympani, to Snooks who sits in the farther corner of a large amphitheater, busily engaged making spitballs for target practice upon the professor's spectacles."[27] But a student's qualifications or his work might play a minor role in determining whether he graduated. Robert M. King, professor at the St. Louis College of Physicians and Surgeons, declared that in order to graduate, the student had to attend "two short terms of four months each," and submit to "a final examination of head and *pocket;* for there is a parting fee of twenty-five dollars demanded for a diploma, which, if written in Latin, not one percent. of the graduates can translate into fair English." The result, then, was that thousands of young medical doctors were "ground out annually," sent forth "to the slaughter of the innocents, as reckless squanderers of drugs and, it may be, as scourges . . . more fearful than pestilence itself."[28]

The situation had not improved, and medicine did not receive the prestige expected of a "learned profession." In 1875 the *New York Daily Tribune* published an editorial quoting Dr. H. C. Wood, the editor of the *Philadelphia Medical Times.* Wood had asserted that the colleges were nothing but "joint-stock companies" that "vie with each other in shortening the time of study and lowering the standard of graduation." He concluded that too many physicians learned medicine after they had been "let loose" to practice "upon the unlucky bodies of the poorer class of patients."[29]

The following year, the *Tribune* editorialized on the work of the American Medical Association and declared that the most important task facing the AMA was to restrict the colleges and prevent the graduation of fraudulent, poorly educated physicians. "A few months' attendance at lectures, a sham examination, and the vulgar quacks, Bob Sawyers, are turned out, thousands at a time, licensed to kill or to cure." Finally in 1879 the *Tribune* came up with the logical conclusion in an editorial entitled "Doctors by Battalions." It exclaimed that the education of physicians was so faulty that it was "a farce to speak of medicine as one of the learned professions."[30]

Some observers concluded that the problem was simply that there were too many colleges. Charles H. Spilman of Kentucky declared: "We could dispense with at least two-thirds of our Medical Colleges, and the remaining ones would be amply sufficient." He recognized that reform was necessary, but he was pessimistic about the chances of ever achieving it. True reform, he said, could come from the government or the colleges themselves. Yet during the Gilded Age it was considered un-American for the government to interfere with business, to regulate admission into a profession, or to meddle with the requirements of the colleges. Reform could also be accomplished by the colleges, but Spilman noted that it would be "suicidal" for any college to initiate reform. He suggested that the medical societies start the reform by accepting only qualified practitioners, in effect making membership in the societies a "badge of superiority."[31]

Even if a few colleges improved over the following years, the general situation grew worse due to a renewed proliferation of the schools. In 1880 there had been ninety colleges, most of them inferior. By 1890 the number of schools had increased to 116. From 1890 to 1900 the number had skyrocketed to 151; by 1906 it had increased by another ten to 161.[32] The result was an even greater number of inferior schools and increased competition among colleges, which made it less likely that reform would ever take place. Ultimately there was a greater likelihood that an increase in the number of inferior schools would result in the production of greater numbers of inferior physicians. More significantly, this proliferation of colleges came precisely when it was becoming more and more difficult for schools to provide a quality medical education.

During the last three decades of the nineteenth century, there had been a scientific revolution in medicine, a revolution that the late Richard H. Shryock, the dean of American medical historians, called "the triumph of modern medicine."[33] The early pathologists had identified specific diseases, which resulted in a revival of interest in parasitology and bacteriology. In 1876 Robert Koch demonstrated that a specific bacterium caused anthrax in animals, and in 1879 Neisser found the gonococcus. In 1881 Pasteur and Sternberg, working independently, described the pneumococcus. Bacteriological developments were coming at a frantic pace. Koch discovered the tubercle bacillus, and in 1883 Klebs and Loeffler found the diphtheria bacillus. In that same year, the "new bacteriology" was to have its first great test. Once again, as it had periodically during the century, cholera threatened to sweep into Europe. Koch, working in Egypt, found a "comma bacillus" associated with the disease. Then he went to India, the seat of the disease, where he managed to isolate the bacillus in culture; he demonstrated that the disease was spread by soiled garments and contaminated water.

Toward the end of the century, the causes of tetanus, typhoid, and bubonic plague were discovered, and similar discoveries were made with malaria, yellow fever, and Texas fever. The importance of preventive medicine was apparent. Mortality rates began to fall, and one by one the horrible scourges of the past began to disappear, either through mass immunization or improved sanitary engineering.

The scientific revolution in medicine increased the importance of chemistry, pathology, bacteriology, and physiology, all of which required intensive laboratory work. Thus the colleges should have been demanding a stronger preliminary education; in order to study physiology, pathology, and bacteriology, it was necessary to have a strong foundation in physics, chemistry, and biology. In addition, with these developments, the teachers could no longer be general practitioners working in their spare time. There was a need for well-trained professors who could devote all of their time to the needs of the students. This meant having endowed medical schools that did not depend upon student fees for support. Yet this was the period when the number of inferior schools multiplied at the greatest rate, making medical reform more urgent than ever before.[34]

A move in the direction of reform came in the 1870s and 1880s when some states began passing medical license laws. For a number of reasons, however, these laws were inadequate. First, the laws were not uniform, and not all states adopted them. This meant that a strong license law in one state would only drive quacks to nearby states that had no regulations. Some states established two or three examining boards in order to protect the homeopaths and eclectics from what they feared would be tyranny of the orthodox practitioners. As a result, in some states each board had its own set of standards. An inadequately prepared applicant might have been licensed by one board, while another board would have rejected the same person. In addition, many of the early laws provided no penalty for practicing without a license. Finally, the laws generally provided for the licensing of every medical graduate without examination.

The problem with the laws can be seen from a letter written by a member of the North Carolina examining board to the state medical journal. In the letter, Dr. Robert Lee Payne complained about the inadequacies of the law. While North Carolina had legislated against carrying concealed weapons, he said, "she allows thousands of mountebanks to scatter broadcast all over the land the *most virulent poisons* in the form of nostrums, which are far more insidious and deadly than the pistol or the dirk." Similarly, the state had erected jails and scaffolds for murderers and other criminals, "yet she permits the most arrant and ignorant quack, who is so inclined, to murder the innocent and ignorant classes of her inhabitants at pleasure." Because there was no penalty for violating the medical license law, virtually anyone could practice medicine in North Carolina.[35]

Payne described the deadly result of ineffective legislation. "Why sir," he said, "I know a man who professes to be a graduate of one of the Baltimore schools (and I expect he is) who was sent for not long since to attend a sick child. After going through the farce of an examination, he gave the poor little thing an ordinary emetic." When that failed to bring about a cure, he "made the father of the child catch some house flies, and after mashing them up with sugar, actually forced the child to swallow them." Payne then told of a "physician" who received a letter from a Baltimore professor, saying that he could enroll in college, "as preparatory study under a preceptor is not necessary." After three months in Baltimore, that same fellow came "back a full-fledged doctor" who was soon "doing considerable practice."[36] Even if he could not pass the medical license examination, he would be penalized only by not being able to sue to collect his fees. The law provided no punishment for murdering patients.

Stanford Chaillé, a New Orleans physician affiliated with the University of Louisiana, made a survey of the medical license legislation in 1879.[37] In the process, he demonstrated the inadequacy of the laws in most states. According to Chaillé, only seven of the thirty-eight states had effective legislation.[38] In Connecticut, there were "no legal restrictions, whatever," and "Connecticut was a paradise of the medical tramp." In Indiana and Iowa, anyone who called himself a doctor could practice medicine. In Kansas, "the most ignorant pretender may dub himself doctor and practice medicine." In Louisiana the tax collector issued licenses on payment of twenty dollars. Chaillé noted that the collector was "so pleased" to receive the fee that he issued the license "without annoying himself further as to the requirements of the law." In Massachusetts "charlatanism infests every city and town," and Missouri was reported to have been "overrun with Quacks."[39]

A note in the *Bulletin of the American Academy of Medicine* perfectly described the reasons for the inadequate laws, at least according to the advocates of reform. It seems that the Ohio legislature defeated a bill to license physicians but at the same time appropriated $5,000 to test the efficacy of the Keeley cure (which employed a totally useless drug and a dry stay at a Keeley spa) for alcoholism. The *Bulletin* declared, "Each member" of the legislature "is to have the privilege of sending one patient to be cured (or of going himself)."[40]

As indicated earlier, the medical license laws often provided that a medical graduate did not have to be examined by the board. Considering the low state of medical education, this provision was ridiculous. By placing a premium on a degree, it encouraged unqualified students to enroll in the colleges, adding to the already devastating competition among medical schools. Then, there was a completely unforeseen development, the growth of medical diploma mills.[41]

Among the earliest diploma mills to develop during this period was the one established in Philadelphia by John Buchanan. In 1853 the Pennsylvania legislature chartered the American College of Medicine; from then to 1870 the college apparently was fairly respectable. But with the license laws putting a premium on the degree, Buchanan sensed a gold mine—thousands of men and women would happily pay for a diploma. Turning the school into a diploma mill was good business; it drastically reduced operating expenses and increased profits. There was no need for laboratories, hospital affiliations, a faculty, and other "frills." The only expense was the cost of operating the printing press.

Buchanan hired agents to search for customers, and they found more than sixty thousand people willing to pay for medical degrees. In 1880 the *Philadelphia Record* gathered evidence against Buchanan. Reporters applied for diplomas and received them by return mail.[42] When the evidence was turned over to the authorities, Buchanan was arrested for using the mails to defraud, violating the law by selling diplomas, and forging the signatures of the so-called professors. After being released on bail, he decided to escape to Canada, but first he faked a drowning in order to save money for his bondsman. Eventually Buchanan was captured and sentenced to a term in prison.[43]

The diploma mills followed the general business practices of the Gilded Age. They hired agents who worked on commission, and they offered a large selection to the customer. For instance, the operator of the Trinity University of Medicine and Surgery of Bennington, Vermont, also sold diplomas from the University of Cincinnati, Montreal Medical College, New York State Medical College, Trenton Medical College, and the University of New Hampshire.[44]

The diploma mills provided would-be physicians with a slightly more respectable alternative to practicing without a diploma, as well as a tremendous saving of time and money compared with the more traditional medical education. The effects of the mills must have been disastrous. When the Illinois Board of Health was given the power to license physicians, it found that from 1877 to 1879 almost 10 percent of the practitioners in the state had purchased their diplomas.[45] The life of the patient was still in danger, not only from the physicians who might have continued to practice heroic medicine, not only from malpractice by practitioners whose education was inadequate, but also from those who simply decided one day to become physicians by purchasing their diplomas.

In spite of the fact that the advocates of medical reform had worked for almost fifty years, the situation in the colleges had grown worse. The schools had continued to proliferate, diploma mills had developed in response to the inadequacies of the license laws, and inferior students were still being admitted to the colleges and turned into physicians.

Notes

1. *Transactions of the American Medical Assocation* 17 (1866): 28, 37.
2. Ibid. 18 (1867): 369-73. See also *Medical Record* 2 (May 15, 1867): 130-133.
3. *Transactions of the AMA* 18 (1867): 381-384.
4. Ibid. 19 (1868): 27-28.
5. Ibid. 32-33.

6. Ibid. 20 (1869): 67-69.

7. Ibid., 77.

8. Ibid., 130-132.

9. Ibid., 34-36.

10. Ibid. 22 (1871): 159-167.

11. *New Orleans Medical and Surgical Journal* 23 (July 1870): 678-684.

12. Quoted in Stanford E. Chaillé, "The Medical Colleges, the Medical Profession, and the Public," *New Orleans Medical and Surgical Journal,* n.s. 1 (May 1874): 823-824.

13. Ibid., 825-829.

14. Ibid., passim.

15. See *Transactions of the AMA* 20 (1869): 30-31; 21 (1870): 37.

16. Ibid. 22 (1871): 12-13.

17. Ibid., 127-128.

18. Ibid., 147.

19. Ibid., 26-27.

20. Henry J. Bigelow, "Medical Education in America," *Medical Communications of the Massachusetts Medical Society* 11 (1874): 235-236.

21. Charles McIntyre, "The Percentage of College-Bred Men in the Medical Profession," *Medical Record* 22 (December 16, 1882): 681-684.

22. L. B. How, *Medical Education* (Manchester, N.H., 1869), pp. 6-8.

23. William W. Green, "Private Preceptorship in the Study of Medicine," *Boston Medical and Surgical Journal* 105 (July 7, 1881): 25-29.

24. Ibid.

25. Ibid. See also Maine Medical Association, *Records of the Twelfth Annual Meeting, 1864-65* (Portland, 1865), pp. 30ff.

26. Isaac A. Abt, *Baby Doctor* (New York and London, 1944), p. 24.

27. W. D. Buck, *Medical Education* (Manchester, N.H., 1869), p. 15.

28. Robert M. King, "Shall We Have a Higher Standard of Medical Education?" *St. Louis Clinical Record* 8 (March 1882): 341-348.

29. *New York Daily Tribune,* November 22, 1875.

30. Ibid., June 10, 1876, March 3, 1879.

31. C. H. Spilman, "The Defects in our Present System of Medical Education," *Kentucky State Medical Society, Transactions, 1872* (Louisville, 1872), p. 75.

32. American Medical Association, Council on Medical Education, *Medical Schools of the United States, 1906* (Chicago, 1906), p. 46.

33. The following paragraphs are derived from Richard H. Shryock, *The Development of Modern Medicine* (New York, 1947), pp. 273ff, 318ff.

34. See N. P. Colwell, "Medical Education," in *U.S. Commissioner of Education, Report, 1915* (Washington, D.C., 1915), 1: 185-220.

35. *North Carolina Medical Journal* 16 (January 1885): 9-10.

36. Ibid., 10-11.

37. Stanford E. Chaillé, "State Medicine and State Medical Societies," *Transactions of the AMA* 30 (1879): 299-355.

38. These were Alabama, California, Illinois, Kentucky, New Hampshire, Texas, Wisconsin, and the District of Columbia. California, Kentucky, and the District of Columbia allowed automatic licensing of graduates.

39. Chaillé, "State Medicine," 327, 331-335, 339, 344.

40. *Bulletin of the American Academy of Medicine* 1 (October 1891): 177.

41. For further information on the medical diploma mills, see Martin Kaufman, "American Medical Diploma Mills," *Bulletin of the Tulane Medical Faculty* 26 (February 1967): 53-57.

42. *Medical and Surgical Reporter* 26 (April 6, 1872): 308-310; *Medical Record* 17 (June 26, 1880): 726-727.

43. *Medical Record* 19 (April 9, 1881): 405.

44. *New York Medical Times* 17 (October 1889): 217-218.

45. See Illinois Board of Health, *Official Register of Physicians and Midwives* (Springfield, 1880), p. 252.

8
Sporadic Improvements

A few colleges did react favorably to the AMA standards of medical education. In the 1840s, the University of Pennsylvania and the College of Physicians and Surgeons had expanded their terms, but faced with competition from colleges that ignored the recommendations, they were forced to revert to the shorter programs.[1] The first college to introduce a permanent reform was Lind University, which became Chicago Medical College and which later affiliated with Northwestern University.

Nathan Smith Davis, a leader in the AMA drive to raise standards of education, played the major role in the development of Lind University. In 1849, as a member of the faculty of the Rush Medical College, Davis argued in favor of revising the program to bring it into line with the AMA proposals. He advocated a graded curriculum, as well as higher standards of preliminary education. When Davis made these suggestions, he encountered vehement opposition from the president of the college, Daniel Brainard, an ambitious surgeon who was convinced that "educational standards must be sacrificed in a free-for-all struggle to attract students." In 1857 while Brainard was in Europe, Davis convinced the faculty to institute the needed reforms. When Brainard discovered what had been done, he rejected the changes, undoubtedly convinced that increased standards would destroy the college by driving away prospective students.[2]

In 1859 the trustees of Lind University in Chicago proposed to establish a medical department and allow the faculty to determine policy. Four physicians agreed to join the faculty, and they invited Davis and a colleague to join them from Rush. Because the college was endowed by Sylvester Lind, it did not have to depend upon student fees, thus enabling Davis to develop a college that could adhere to the AMA standards. In 1863 a business failure prevented Lind from continuing to support the school, and the professors were forced to strike out on their own; they formed the Chicago Medical College.[3]

By 1880 their school provided medical training superior to that of Rush Medical College, their major competitor. While Rush continued to admit all who applied, Chicago Medical College required students either to be college graduates or to undergo an examination by the faculty to ascertain that they had a good preliminary education. Because the students at Chicago Medical College took a five-month graded course, compared with the shorter and more traditional program at Rush, many more students matriculated at the latter school. In 1880 Rush could boast of an enrollment of 440, while the reformed college had only 148 students. In addition, since Chicago had a larger faculty, Rush was far more profitable for each professor. It was especially profitable when one considers that the term at Rush was a full month shorter than at Chicago Medical College.[4]

From its founding in 1859 to 1870, the Chicago Medical College stood alone in opposition to the destructive competition, striving to maintain high standards in spite of a decreased enrollment and reduced compensation of the faculty.[5] The next significant reform came at a most unlikely place, Harvard Medical College, which earlier had so vehemently opposed the medical reforms advocated by the AMA. When Charles Eliot became president of Harvard University, the medical college was "essentially a proprietary school, with a curriculum of four months of lectures during each of two years." In addition to attendance at lectures, students were required to spend eight months as apprentices to practicing physicians or as house officers at either Massachusetts General or Boston City Hospital.[6]

The students had to pass final examinations, which amounted to little more than a ridiculous game of musical tables. Nine students were examined at one time. They entered a large room containing nine professors, each at his own table. The students stopped for five minutes at each table, answering questions posed by the professors. After the five minutes had elapsed, Henry Bigelow rang a bell and the students went to the next table. In forty-five minutes, when the examination ended for those students, they all left the room. Then Bigelow would call the name of a student and each professor would hold up a card. If the student had satisfactorily answered the questions, the professor would hold the card white side up. If he failed, the card would show a black ball. If a student received five white cards, he would receive a degree. This meant that a student could get a Harvard medical degree even if he could not answer one question in four branches of medical science.[7] It was especially farcical when we consider examining a student in a five-minute period. James Clarke White, who later became a member of the faculty, said that his examination in surgery consisted of one question: "Well, White, what would you do for a wart?"[8]

Eliot became convinced of the need for improving the medical college. He reported that "the whole system of medical education . . . needs thorough reformation." The president of the board of overseers, Charles Francis Adams, agreed with Eliot, describing how a recent Harvard Medical School graduate had killed three men by overdoses of morphine. Eliot's drive for reform split the faculty into two factions. On one side were the younger liberals who advocated reform, on the other Henry Bigelow and Oliver Wendell Holmes. Holmes reversed his position when the movement to reform the college gathered steam.[9]

Bigelow was clearly the leader of the opposition. He devoted a great deal of time and energy defending the existing system of medical education at Harvard. Physicians were born and not trained, he said, which meant that a reduction in the number of students would diminish the possibility of training the great ones. In 1871 when Bigelow spoke before the Massachusetts Medical Society, he made specific reference to the proposed changes at Harvard: "You cannot turn out medical men with the uniform perfection of Ames shovels or Springfield muskets," he declared, also noting that no school could afford "on any ground to lose sight of the size of its classes, which are at once the seed and its fertilizer."[10]

Finally, Eliot told the faculty that debate was useless; the Harvard

Corporation had decided to carry out the changes, regardless of opposition. Bigelow was obviously outraged that the decision was being made by laymen. "Does Mr. Lowell know anything about Medical education?" he asked, "or Reverend Putnam? or Judge Bigelow? Why," he exclaimed, "Mr. Crowninshield carries a horse-chestnut in his pocket to keep off rheumatism!" Bigelow asked rhetorically whether the "new medical education" would be "best directed by a man who carries horse-chestnuts in his pockets to cure rheumatism." When Eliot suggested requiring written examination for graduation, Bigelow responded that Eliot "knew nothing about the quality of the Harvard medical students; more than half of them can barely write. Of course, they can't pass written examinations."[11]

In 1871, in spite of the opposition, Harvard announced a thorough reformation: a three-year course of studies, a graded curriculum, a nine-month term, and oral and written examinations in every department. Albeit unwillingly, Harvard had followed the lead of Chicago Medical College. The dire predictions of Bigelow and others proved correct. From 1870 to 1872 Harvard's enrollment decreased by 43 percent.[12] Students simply did not want to spend nine months in each of three years learning medicine; it was possible to attend other schools for four months in two years and receive the same type of degree.

In 1877 the University of Pennsylvania, with William Pepper taking the lead, followed Harvard in developing a three-year graded curriculum. The faculty was satisfied with fixed salaries, which no longer made them dependent on student demands for quick and easy degrees.[13] Chicago, Harvard, and Pennsylvania were followed by Syracuse and Michigan; the movement to reform medical education received its first positive boost from an enlightened group of colleges.

In 1877 the drive was given renewed strength by the successful movement to regulate medicine in Illinois. As medical licensure and reform went hand in hand, this could do nothing but demonstrate the advantages offered by the superior colleges. The Illinois legislature established a state board of health and gave it the power to enforce the medical practice law. In order to practice medicine legally, all physicians had to register with the board of health. By law, the board had to license all who had practiced in the state for more than ten years. All others were required to present a diploma from a medical college or they had to undergo an examination by the state board of health.

The governor appointed three orthodox physicians to the board, along with one homeopath, one eclectic, and two laymen who were leading educators. Almost immediately John H. Rauch, one of the orthodox physicians, became the dominant force on the board, and he gained the title "the John the Baptist of reform" for his zealous work to improve medical practice in Illinois. The Illinois law went into effect on July 1, 1877, and the board began to issue licenses. Its 1878 report indicated that a total of 4,950 physicians had been granted licenses to practice medicine. These included 3,858 who were certified on possession of their diplomas, 942 on ten years' practice, and 150 on passing the examination. Rauch reported that about 1,400 practitioners had left Illinois when the law went into effect, and of the 371 nongraduates who were examined, only 150 passed.[14] This meant that almost 25 percent of the practitioners in Illinois were either rejected by the board or left the state rather than submit to examination.

The board also registered midwives, with similar results. Almost half of the practicing midwives in Illinois were unqualified. Before the passage of the licensing act, there had been about 856 midwives in the state. About 300 of those stopped practicing in 1877 and 1878. Of those who were licensed, 132 possessed diplomas and licenses, mostly issued by foreign schools and organizations. The board licensed 376 on the basis of ten years' practice, and 58 were registered after passing an examination administered by the board of health.[15]

The Illinois board uncovered a great deal of evidence that diplomas were being sold and that diploma mills were in active operation. In its first report, the board noted that about 400 diplomas were held by people "who had either bought them directly, or obtained them upon a nominal examination. Agencies of these diploma-shops were found in different parts of the state, and for a time," the board reported, "the sale of diplomas was pressed with considerable vigor under the impression that the Board would recognize them." The board noted that fraudulent diplomas were possessed by "nearly all the vilest professional mountebanks, and the advertising specialists, quacks and abortionists," as well as those who travelled "from town to town, promising to cure all the ailments that flesh is heir to." Interestingly, the report noted that the diploma mills produced degrees that were "works of art"; they were "more imposing and exceed in style" the diplomas issued by the regular colleges.[16]

On November 15, 1877, the board decided that it had to take more positive action in order to ensure a high level of medical care in the state. It was determined to raise the level of medical education, in Illinois at least, by refusing to recognize the diploma of any school that offered two courses in the same year and that did not require two courses of lectures for graduation.[17]

In 1881 the board established a subcommittee to investigate the conditions in the various colleges and to report on what constituted a college "in good standing." The committee did a great deal of research, even to the extent of sending queries to every medical college in the country and requesting information from the leading medical societies. After studying eighty-seven replies, the committee reported that although it would be satisfying to set high standards, that would not be practical due to the small number of good colleges. Minimum standards *were* established, however, and everyone applying for a license to practice in Illinois had to submit a diploma from a college that fulfilled the board's requirements.

In order to be approved, a college had to require students to document their "adequate" preparatory education by being either college graduates or products of good high schools or by undergoing a thorough examination by the faculty. Furthermore, no college could be certified unless it required students to have a minimum of three years of total study, including a two-year college course that included dissection and clinical and hospital instruction. The board concluded by noting the absurdity of a system that expected "to make skillful physicians of illiterate students, by mere dint of reading them lectures, even when accompanied by quizzes and examinations."[18]

In 1881 more evidence was found that a number of diploma mills were blatantly operating in Illinois and elsewhere. One case began when "Dr." J. B. Thompson of Chicago applied for a license to practice medicine. He presented a diploma from the Bellevue Medical College of Massachusetts, a school that the board had not approved. When the board investigated, there seemed to be indications that the "college" was a diploma mill. To learn the truth, the board had a young journalist, V. B. Kelly, write for a "diplomy." In his letter, he said that he had "bin Redin medesin about a year." The proprietor of the college, Rufus King Noyes of Lynn, responded by offering a diploma for $150 if Kelly could submit a short dissertation. Kelly sent a thesis on "Vacination," in which he demonstrated an inability to spell, a total unawareness of the rules of punctuation, and a lack of medical knowledge. Noyes informed him by mail that his thesis had been examined "by the Professors and found to be acceptable." The diploma was sent COD.[19]

These discoveries focused public attention on the diploma mill scandals. The realization that mills existed throughout the country led physicians, legislators, and interested citizens in other states to discuss the need for improving their licensing laws. This came at a time when medicine was becoming more solidly based on valid scientific knowledge. As Richard Shryock indicated, "the wonders of science" were so impressive to the layman that the physician and surgeon once more became respectable. The hospital was changing dramatically, as visible evidence of the "wonders of science." It was transforming from the "pest-house" of the past to the palace of healing of the future. The "striking discoveries in therapeutics and preventive medicine, and the resulting decline in mortality, were bound to impress the public."[20] As the public attitude toward physicians and medicine became more favorable and as medical practice became more firmly based on science, physicians were able to put up a stronger case for regulation.

At the same time, two other developments in the same direction were taking place. One was the establishment of the American Academy of Medicine, with membership limited to those physicians who had graduated from college before enrolling in medical school. This was intended to make a distinction between the average doctor, who was poorly educated, and the top-flight physician who possessed the qualifications and the training for successful scientific medical practice.[21] A second and related movement was the formation of the American Medical College Association, which was similar to earlier attempts to initiate reform of medical education through cooperation

of several schools. The association developed out of a convention of
professors in June 1876, which was called by a committee led by John
B. Biddle of Jefferson Medical College.

Before the convention could meet, however, the problems it
would encounter were demonstrated in an open letter to Biddle from
seven faculty members of the Kentucky School of Medicine. The
letter began by condemning preliminary education examinations as
"quixotic," deceptive, and to the advantage of those colleges that
advocated them. The Kentucky professors declared that "the greatest blessings to medical science have been derived from those who
entered the profession comparatively uneducated." They concluded:
"We can neither deprive the Profession of similar blessings in
future," nor close "the doors to a useful and often distinguished
career" upon those who had been "deprived of early education."[22]

The teachers expressed their opposition to the graduation fee,
arguing that it was tantamount to "selling diplomas" and that it placed
the professor in the position "that an affirmative vote brings him
money, while a negative vote deprives him of it." Now that they had
placed themselves on firm moral grounds, the Kentucky faculty
declared that they fully supported the "AMA rule" that urged colleges to charge $120 for tuition. "We announce ourselves," they said,
"ready to observe, in good faith, the very highest tuition fees adopted
by the majority of the convention."[23]

Finally, the faculty at Kentucky advocated the practice of awarding
"beneficiary" scholarships to needy students. They asserted that the
scholarship was necessary for the high-fee colleges "surrounded by
low-fee schools." If aid were not offered, there would be a massive
rush to enroll in the low-fee institutions.[24]

In spite of its moral stance, the Kentucky School of Medicine was
one of the most flagrant offenders. In an interesting arrangement,
the college had the same faculty as the Louisville Medical College.
Since it was considered unprofessional to offer two courses in the
same year, the Louisville Medical College held its term in the fall,
and students and faculty alike transferred to the Kentucky School of
Medicine in spring. In that way the students completed their studies
in one year, the professors collected fees for two terms, and the
faculty exclaimed that it had "reformed" by its refusal to offer two
terms a year in the same college.[25]

In any case, in June 1876 the delegates to the Philadelphia convention gathered once again to discuss the problem of medical education. Also once again, the delegates represented a minority of the total number of colleges. The schools that were represented, however, were quite diverse. Delegates came from the large urban schools like the Jefferson Medical College and New York's College of Physicians and Surgeons. Some small proprietary colleges were represented, such as the Long Island Hospital Medical College, the Starling Medical College of Ohio, and the Keokuk College of Physicians and Surgeons. Delegates came from the state medical college of Iowa, and a number of schools with college and university affiliation were represented, including the University of Georgia, the University of Pennsylvania, Vanderbilt University, the University of Vermont, and Syracuse University.[26] Except for the University of Vermont, no New England schools were represented.

The delegates elected John Biddle as president, and Leartus Connor of the Detroit Medical College became secretary. A committee was appointed to submit items for consideration. Perhaps the most significant item on the agenda was the question as to whether the association should be made permanent. After debate, it was decided that the association should not be allowed to disappear like its predecessors, and the professors voted that this first gathering would be considered the "Provisional" Association of American Medical Colleges.[27]

The delegates discussed whether they should condemn or endorse the beneficiary system, "with its present abuses." As indicated above, some colleges had been giving scholarships to large numbers of students as a way to fill empty benches and in order to attract students who otherwise might have attended competing schools. The colleges that offered "beneficiaries" expected at least to break even by collecting enrollment and graduation fees from every student. The delegates decided that the indiscriminate use of the system was unjust and that it should not be condoned except in "unusual cases."

Another item under consideration was whether there should be a minimum time period between enrollment and graduation. This was necessary in order to prevent students from attending two different colleges and graduating nine months after having started their medical studies. The association decided that no college should be allowed to graduate any student who had enrolled for his first course of lectures during the same year, and it was agreed that there must be a fifteen-month period between the time a student entered medical college and the time he graduated.

The delegates voted in favor of a graded curriculum, decided to retain graduation fees, and finally announced that since homeopathy was quackery, homeopathic colleges could not send representatives to future conventions. The first meeting of the Association of American Medical Colleges represented an excellent start. The question, however, was whether the colleges would agree to reform themselves and whether the association could enforce its standards.

In 1878 the organization, then called the American Medical College Assocation, refused to recognize the Nashville Medical College, which offered two graduating courses in one year and considered three years of practice as the equivalent of one course of lectures. In an important move, Samuel D. Gross of the Jefferson Medical College suggested that the association adopt a uniform system of instruction, and it was agreed that the delegates would be prepared to discuss this prior to the 1879 AMA convention.[28]

In 1879 the convention began with the announcement that due to an inability to lengthen its course to twenty weeks, Dartmouth withdrew from the association. Next the delegates debated whether it was possible to require a preliminary examination and whether it was feasible to demand a three-year course of studies. Although the delegates voted in favor of both ideas, they decided that no binding action should be taken until the articles of confederation of the association could be amended. At that point, it was moved to amend the articles to read that a member college had to require a three-year course of study. The motion was tabled for one year to allow for thorough discussion by the individual faculties.[29]

Samuel D. Gross was "bitterly disappointed" when the meeting adjourned without reaching a significant decision on the matter. He declared in his autobiography: "Alas, two entire days were spent in idle, vapid talk," and he exclaimed that the convention ended "like its two predecessors, in smoke."[30]

His disappointment was to be compounded by developments at the 1880 meeting of the association. The delegates voted twenty to nothing in favor of requiring a three-year course of study, but the

Jefferson Medical College had apparently decided against that change; the delegate from Jefferson did not cast his ballot on the issue. Next it was announced that three colleges were withdrawing from the association—New York's College of Physicians and Surgeons, the Bellevue Hospital Medical College, and the University of Vermont.

When Secretary Leartus Connor presented his report of the meeting, he credited the association with having made significant improvements in medical education. He declared that the association had diminished the number of diplomas bestowed without study and examination and had reduced the number of "dead heads" in the schools. Furthermore, Connor said that the association's rule against reduction of fees had eliminated the "undignified bidding for students" and thus increased respect for the colleges. Of course, an end to "beneficiary" scholarships resulted in an increase of income for the colleges, in addition. Connor emphasized the fact that the standards of the association had been adopted by nearly all the colleges that had been organized during the past five years. Finally, except for the University of Virginia and Harvard, all the colleges that had previously offered two courses in one year had abandoned that practice.[31]

In 1880 N. S. Davis and Samuel D. Gross submitted a committee report to the American Medical College Association in which they lambasted the Harvard faculty for its disregard of the demand for thorough reform. They noted that students at Harvard could be granted advanced standing by passing an examination, and they declared: "He must be a rather dull young man" who could not convince a physician to be his preceptor, take the necessary books, and in two years learn enough to pass the Harvard examination for two years' advanced standing. The report pointed out that Harvard "is today offering her diploma for a less amount of medical college attendance and instruction than any other respectable school in this country." Davis and Gross concluded by declaring that although Harvard's faculty had received a great deal of publicity when it announced a fourth year, since it was optional, very few students would bother to take advantage of it.[32]

Perhaps Connor's enthusiasm for the cause of reform can be seen in the changes made at his school, the Detroit Medical College. In 1879, after the association had urged a graded curriculum, the

Detroit college developed a "voluntary" system that allowed students to take sequential courses. A year later, after the association had voted in favor of a three-year curriculum, the college required students to attend for three full years and by then the "voluntary" graded curriculum had become mandatory.[33]

Yet in spite of Connor's obvious zeal, the association was about to face its greatest threat. A definite split was developing between the larger eastern colleges and the association, which to a large extent represented schools in the West and South. For instance, New York's *Medical Record* editorialized on the achievements of the association and declared that it had "failed utterly" in its attempt to set minimum fees and that it had not stopped underbidding. In addition the *Medical Record* noted that although clinical work was a requirement for membership in the association, a "good many" country schools could not possibly enforce this because of a lack of adequate hospital facilities. The editorial concluded: "The country colleges should accept the fact that their function in medical education is a limited one, and they should be content with the position of a lower grade college."[34]

The *Chicago Medical Journal and Examiner* responded to the attack of the *Medical Record.* In an editorial probably written by N. S. Davis, who was on the editorial staff, the Chicago journal noted that the eastern cities did not have the largest colleges. Rush Medical College in Chicago was larger than any eastern school, and the total number of students in Chicago, Cincinnati, St. Louis, Louisville, and New Orleans was equal to that attending schools in Philadelphia, New York City, Brooklyn, and Boston. In addition, since the American Medical College Association had been established, no college offered less than a two-year course of study and the Louisville problem had been eliminated. Moreover, all the colleges in the association had increased their fees except for the state universities of Michigan and Iowa, where tuition was determined by state law.[35]

The editorial suggested that perhaps the College of Physicians and Surgeons and the Bellevue Hospital Medical College had helped establish the association in the hope of drawing in New York University, which offered scholarships to every student, expecting the fees and a large student body to make up the difference. Because the university had not joined the organization, it was difficult for the other two schools to compete and remain members of the association. The editorial noted that Dartmouth withdrew because it was threatened by the rule requiring fifteen months between enrollment and graduation. Many students attended Dartmouth because its term ended in time for the start of the courses in Boston and New York City; thus, students could take a second course, finishing their degrees in nine months of medical study. In the next issue of the *Chicago Medical Journal and Examiner,* the same editorialist angrily declared that he was impatient at the "Pecksniffian assumption that there is nothing of value or importance in the medical institutions of the country outside of that circumscribed strip of territory lying between the eastern part of the Alleghanies and Plymouth Rock."[36]

Meanwhile, eleven colleges resigned from the association. They were unwilling to institute a three-year course, fearing competition from colleges that were not members of the organization.[37] In a signed editorial by N. S. Davis, the Chicago journal complained that the colleges in the "great Eastern cities" were always playing "dog in the manger, each for itself," while they tried to make the "so-called 'smaller colleges scattered throughout the West and South,' the *scape-goats* for the sins that are pre-eminently their own."[38] Yet the list of withdrawing institutions indicates that the failure of the association to enforce its reforms could not be blamed on any specific group of schools. Rather, the fact that so many colleges never joined the association was a major influence. It was difficult, if not impossible, to reform when nonmember institutions would benefit from the increased standards of their competition.

At its 1882 meeting, the remaining members of the American Medical College Association decided to take a step backward in order to remain in existence. Member schools were authorized to consider two sessions of five months each as equivalent to three courses of study. This is precisely what was instituted at Detroit Medical College in spite of Leartus Connor's enthusiasm for reform. The three-year course had resulted in such a decline in enrollment that the survival of the college was threatened. In 1883 the college granted degrees after only two years of study.[39]

The retreat from its earlier moral stance was hardly sufficient to save the association. The fact that it was forced to withdraw from its crusade destroyed the incentive of those who had remained in the association. As a result, no meetings of the organization were held from 1882 to 1889.[40]

Notes

1. See above, pp. 102-103.

2. Thomas N. Bonner, "Dr. Nathan Smith Davis and the Growth of Chicago Medicine, 1850-1900," *Bulletin of the History of Medicine* 26 (July-August 1952): 363ff. See also I. N. Danforth, *Life of Nathan Smith Davis* (Chicago, 1907), p. 18.

3. Bonner, "Dr. Nathan Smith Davis," 363ff.; N. S. Davis, "The Earlier History of the Medical School," in Arthur H. Wilde, ed., *Northwestern University: A History* (New York, 1905), 3: 298-308.

4. E. Fletcher Ingals, "A Review of the Progress of Medical Education in Chicago," *Chicago Medical Journal and Examiner* 42 (February 1881): 136-147.

5. The Boston University Medical School was established with entrance examinations and a three-year course in 1873, and in 1874 the faculty voted to let state medical societies examine its students and recommend conferral of degrees. This school, however, was homeopathic, and the homeopathic colleges played a minor role in the mainstream of American medical education. BU's actions were virtually ignored by orthodox colleges and journals. See *New York Daily Tribune,* March 29, 1879, for a survey of the school's medical programs.

6. David Cheever, "The Turn of the Century—and After," *New England Journal of Medicine* 222: 1-11, quoted in John F. Fulton, *Harvey Cushing: A Biography* (Springfield, Illinois, 1946), p. 55.

7. Joseph C. Aub and Ruth K. Hapgood, *Pioneer in Modern Medicine* (Cambridge, Massachusetts, 1970), pp. 141-142.

8. James Clarke White, *Sketches from My Life: 1833-1913* (Cambridge, Massachusetts, 1914), p. 152.

9. Thomas F. Harrington, *The Harvard Medical School* (Chicago and New York, 1905), 3: 1020-1022; Edward D. Churchill, ed., *To Work in the Vineyard of Surgery: Reminiscences of J. Collins Warren* (Cambridge, Massachusetts, 1958), p. 179. For Holmes's comments, see John T. Morse, *Life and Letters of Oliver Wendell Holmes* (Boston and New York, 1897), 1: 185, 2: 190-191.

10. Harrington, *Harvard Medical School,* 3: 1022, 1029-1032.

11. Quoted in Aub and Hapgood, *Pioneer in Modern Medicine,* p. 141. See also Harrington, *Harvard Medical School,* 3: 1043.

12. Harrington, *Harvard Medical School,* 3: 1057.

13. For details, see William Pepper, *Higher Medical Education* (Philadelphia, 1894), pp. 35-36; Fred B. Rogers, "William Pepper, 1843-1898," *Journal of Medical Education* 34 (September 1959): 885-889; Francis Newton Thorpe, *William Pepper, M.D., LL.D.* (Philadelphia and London, 1940), and George Corner, *Two Centuries of Medicine* (Philadelphia, 1965).

14. H. O. Johnson, "The Regulations of Medical Practice by State Boards of Health," *Transactions of the American Medical Association* 30 (1879): 293-298. See also Illinois State Board of Health, *Annual Report, 1878* (Springfield, 1879), pp. 6-7.

15. Illinois State Board of Health, *Official Register of Physicians and Midwives* (Springfield, 1880), p. 252.

16. Illinois State Board of Health, *Annual Report, 1878,* pp. 16-17.

17. Ibid., p. 18.

18. *Chicago Medical Review* 3 (February 20, 1881): 85-88.

19. *Chicago Medical Times* 14 (December 1882): 421-428; *Journal of the American Medical Association* 23 (July 14, 1894): 83-84. See also Illinois State Board of Health, *Fourth Annual Report, 1882* (Springfield, 1882), pp. xiii-xv; John Rauch to John Shaw Billings, Springfield, Illinois, January 8, 1881, Billings Papers, National Library of Medicine, Bethesda, Maryland.

20. For this development, see chapter 9 below. See also Richard H. Shryock, *The Development of Modern Medicine* (New York, 1947), pp. 336ff.

21. See *Transactions of the AMA* 22 (1871): 28-29; 23 (1872): 45-46.

22. *American Medical Weekly* (Louisville) 4 (June 3, 1876): 364-368.

23. Ibid. There was no such "AMA rule."

24. Ibid.

25. See *Louisville Medical News* 1 (January 1, 1876): 1-3.

26. *Medical Record* 11 (July 1, 1876): 432-434. For a chronological history of the association, see Dean F. Smiley, "History of the Association of American Medical Colleges, 1876-1956," *Journal of Medical Education* 32 (July 1957): 512-525.

27. The following account of this meeting is developed from the two works cited in note 26 and American Association of Medical Colleges, *History of Its Organization* (Detroit, 1877).

28. American Medical College Association, *Proceedings, 1878* (Detroit, 1878), pp. 7-8.

29. Ibid., *1879* (Detroit, 1879), pp. 8-11.

30. *Autobiography of Samuel D. Gross* (Philadelphia, 1887), 2: 70-71.

31. American Medical College Association, *Proceedings, 1880* (Detroit, 1880), pp. 6-10; *Detroit Lancet*, n.s. 4 (July 1880): 36-40.

32. *Chicago Medical Journal and Examiner* 41 (August 1880): 207, 210.

33. See Leslie Hanawalt, *A Place of Light* (Detroit, 1968), pp. 53-55.

34. *Medical Record* 18 (August 14, 1880): 184-185.

35. *Chicago Medical Journal and Examiner* 41 (October 1880): 396-403.

36. Ibid. (November 1880): 504.

37. For a list of the schools withdrawing from the association, see Dean F. Smiley, "History of the American Association of Medical Colleges," *Journal of Medical Education* 32 (July 1957): 514.

38. *Chicago Medical Journal and Examiner* 42 (January 1881): 74-75.

39. Hanawalt, *A Place of Light,* pp. 54-55. See also "President T. A. McGraw's Annual Address to Faculty, Fall, 1889," in Alumni Secretary's Scrapbook number 1, Wayne State University Archives.

40. See American Medical College Association, *Proceedings, 1882* (Detroit, 1882), passim.

9

The Reformers Gain Allies

Developments in medical licensure were crucial for the advancement of American medical education. From the 1840s to the 1870s, in the absence of medical legislation, the nation was virtually overrun with quacks. When the movement to license physicians resumed in the 1870s, the laws provided for the automatic licensing of anyone who possessed a diploma. By placing a premium on the degree, the laws encouraged an extensive traffic in diplomas. It was not long before the glaring loophole that existed was recognized, and physicians and legislators worked to amend the laws to provide for examination of *all* applicants for medical licenses.[1] In 1888 only five states required such examinations; by 1896 eighteen others had amended their laws in the same way.[2]

One way to understand the implications of the changes in medical licensure is to investigate the process by which one state developed effective legislation. New York is an ideal example; sources are available that describe how the state passed through virtually every phase—from the absence of legislation after 1844 to one of the most advanced laws in 1907.[3]

In 1844 the New York State legislature repealed its medical license law. The following years saw a great deal of discussion within the profession. Leading physicians sought to restore order out of the

143

chaos that existed in the absence of effective medical legislation. Finally, in 1874, after a great deal of lobbying by medical interests, a law was passed that required registration of all practitioners. That was a beginning, but the law was totally ineffective. Uneducated "physicians" could continue to practice, and anyone who claimed competence could register as a practitioner without having to undergo an examination.[4]

The inadequacy of the law was obvious to members of the profession as well as to those with an interest in protecting the public from unskilled practitioners. The orthodox physicians prescribed a remedy—a medical examining board to test every applicant for a medical license. Given the mistrust that existed between the allopaths and the unorthodox practitioners, this proposal was bitterly condemned as a "plot" by the American Medical Association to destroy competition. In June 1885 the American Institute of Homeopathy adopted a resolution denouncing the AMA for its attempt to control licensing, and the assembled homeopaths declared their opposition to any legislation that would allow allopaths to examine homeopaths.[5] The homeopaths demanded "equal representation, three separate boards, or nothing."[6]

At this point, the general consensus among the unorthodox physicians was that the government ought to stay out of medical affairs. George W. Winterburn, for instance, the editor of the *American Homeopath,* declared that "every man has the right to employ any other man to do any thing for him, whether it be to take care of his horse or his health. . . . We would not submit to legislative enactment compelling us to patronize John, the butcher, and Dick, the baker," he concluded, "and we see no reason why they should be compelled to have a doctor endorsed by government." Winterburn proposed that physicians abide by the same law as businessmen: "survival of the fittest." The capable physicians would attract enough patients to earn a living, while the unsuccessful ones would be forced to find some other occupation.[7]

By 1889, however, a number of physicians came to recognize that legislation was necessary to protect the public health and safety. Yet in order to ensure passage the orthodox and unorthodox sects had to unite behind the same proposal. Since the irregulars would not trust the allopaths to honestly and objectively evaluate homeopathic practitioners, the only possible solution was the establishment of three separate boards of examiners, one for each sect. William Osler, professor of medicine at Johns Hopkins, declared in 1889 that if the orthodox practitioners really wanted to enact medical license laws, they had to forget the past and unite with the irregulars. Osler recognized that "this is gall and wormwood to many," as a great many allopaths considered homeopathy and eclecticism as legalized quackery. Yet, "in the interest of the public," he suggested that the profession "bury animosities and agree to differ on the question of Therapeutics."[8]

Finally in 1891 that harmony was achieved in New York. After almost twenty years of discussion and debate, the state's medical license law went into effect. The regents of the state university were directed to establish three separate boards of medical examiners, and they appointed board members from lists of those nominated by the three state medical societies: orthodox, homeopathic, and eclectic. The regents developed the examination questions; all applicants would have the same questions in anatomy, surgery, physiology, and the other basic medical fields. Questions in therapeutics would be "in harmony with the tenets of the school selected by the candidate." After September 1891, no one in New York could practice without a license from the regents, and such licenses would only be granted on recommendation of one of the three medical examining boards.[9]

In an interesting development that perhaps indicates the caliber of the medical student of the day, one thousand medical students united in an unsuccessful attempt to exempt the first year "Baby Students" from having to pass an examination upon graduation.[10]

The early years of the three-board system in New York proved to be quite encouraging. In 1894 the orthodox board rejected 32.7 percent, the homeopathic board failed 22 percent, and the eclectic board refused to license 57.1 percent of those examined. Each faction obviously set high standards for those who would henceforth advertise themselves as allopaths, homeopaths, or eclectics.[11] In spite of the apparent success of the system, the orthodox profession was not satisfied. Those allopaths who still considered the irregulars as quacks were convinced that the system legalized quackery by allowing homeopaths and eclectics to appear before their own boards of examiners. Nothing could be done, however, unless it could be proven that the irregulars were licensing incompetents.

Around the turn of the century, the licensing system faced a distinct challenge when newer unorthodox sects appeared on the scene and demanded their own medical licensing boards. Since homeopaths and eclectics were examined by members of their own groups, the osteopaths and Christian Scientists refused to appear before allopathic, homeopathic, or eclectic boards. They demanded the right to have their own licensing boards, which was a logical request considering the existing situation in the state. Yet if the Christian Scientists and osteopaths were successful, the fragmentation of the power to license would have destroyed the system. The *New York Times* insisted, "One Board Is Enough." It noted that if the existing sects did not consolidate the examining boards, the osteopaths and the Christian Scientists would soon have their own examining boards, which would reduce the "whole State licensing system . . . to a farce" and would destroy "the public's protection from quacks."[12]

As a result of the threat to the existing sects, the homeopaths, eclectics, and allopaths in New York united behind a single examining board; a bill to that effect was signed into law in 1907 by Governor Charles Evans Hughes. The new board was composed of nine members representative of the allopaths, homeopaths, and eclectics in proportion to their numbers. In the future, every graduate of a four-year medical course of studies who wanted to practice in New York would have to pass an examination administered by this board. In order to protect the irregulars, there were to be no questions on materia medica or therapeutics. In effect this meant that osteopaths who had taken four-year courses could present themselves for examination. That allowed the older sects to evaluate the abilities of men and women they considered to be quacks.[13] One result, however, was a perceptible improvement in the quality of osteopathy in New York, as it was an incentive for osteopathic colleges to develop thorough four-year courses of study.

Similar developments took place in state after state.[14] By 1896 twenty-three states required examination prior to licensing; sixteen of those states had a unified board of examiners, four had two separate boards, and three had three separate boards. The trend was clearly toward unified boards of examiners.[15]

Even though the states were moving toward more stringent medical licensing examinations, the boards could not be unrealistic in their standards. The fact was that relatively few colleges were providing high-quality medical education. To a large extent, what was needed was an example of the value of a superior medical training. If it could be proven that a college could increase standards without destroying its lifeblood, the flow of students, other schools might initiate similar reforms. After all, America's medical professors were undoubtedly well-intentioned men and women who were realistic in their adherence to a traditional system, especially when reform threatened to be suicidal. Johns Hopkins University was to provide that needed example.

Johns Hopkins was a banker and the largest stockholder in the Baltimore and Ohio Railroad. According to one source he was impressed by the philanthropic work of George Peabody, the London financier who had used his fortune to support educational reform.[16] Just prior to his death in 1873, Hopkins established a board of trustees with instructions to construct a hospital that would "compare favorably with any other institution of like character in this country or Europe." The philanthropist hoped that it might ultimately form the nucleus of a great medical school that would carry his name for posterity. In 1875 the trustees selected five physicians to advise them in planning what was to become the Johns Hopkins Hospital. The advisers included John Shaw Billings of the United States Army, Joseph Jones, who had been active in the National Board of Health, and Stephen Smith, a prominent New York surgeon and public health reformer. The physicians presented individual reports on the construction of a teaching hospital; Billings combined the reports into one workable plan.[17]

Meanwhile, in accordance with Johns Hopkins' will, a university was established. In 1876 the trustees selected Daniel Coit Gilman, president of the University of California, to become president of the newly created Johns Hopkins University.[18] When the trustees approved Billings' plan, construction of the hospital began. At that point, Billings set out to provide the framework for the development of a medical school that would be affiliated with the university and closely interrelated with the hospital. Billings' plans were quite advanced, as well they might be, considering that the school's endowment would make it independent of student fees and pressures. He proposed a four-year graded curriculum which included extensive use of preclinical laboratories and a thorough integration of the work of the college and the teaching hospital.

Some colleges had already started to move in those directions. Harvard already had a preclinical laboratory in physiology, and the University of Pennsylvania and the University of Michigan offered clinical work in a teaching hospital. But Hopkins had the advantage of not having to worry about obstacles erected by local traditions or feelings of the faculty. Significantly, the faculty at Johns Hopkins was to be composed of graduates of the pathfinding universities of Pennsylvania and Michigan.[19]

Billings helped to attract a corps of young faculty, none of whom was over forty and all of whom were familiar with the most recent scientific developments in America and abroad. William Henry Welch, a professor of pathology, had established the first American laboratory in the teaching of microscopic pathology at the Bellevue Hospital Medical College. He had revolutionized the teaching of pathology by emphasizing the use of the laboratory rather than the traditional didactic lectures and recitation based on texts.[20] Indeed, Welch's position at Johns Hopkins was in itself innovative; he was to be a full-time professor rather than a practicing physician who taught pathology on the side. Welch's pathology laboratory was to produce young and enthusiastic scientists such as Walter Reed, who in a short time was to take the lead in the battle against epidemic tropical disease, and Simon Flexner, who was to organize the Rockefeller Institute for Medical Research.[21]

William Osler, who had been professor of medicine at McGill University and at the University of Pennsylvania, was appointed professor of the theory and practice of medicine and physician-in-chief of the Johns Hopkins Hospital. Osler's European training and innovative temperament were to be vital to the success of Johns Hopkins. His conviction that traditional medical education included too little bedside teaching led him to bring third- and fourth-year medical students into the wards as clinical clerks. Osler also introduced the German residency system for advanced training of medical graduates.[22] This was the first organized plan to provide medical students with extensive medical practice prior to and after graduation, and it was revolutionary.

William S. Halsted was appointed professor of surgery, and he proved to be of the same innovative mold as Osler. Like the professor of medicine, he used students in the hospital as surgical dressers, giving advanced students the practical training lacking in traditional medical education.[23] Welch, Halsted, and Osler were joined by Howard Kelly in obstetrics and Franklin B. Mall in anatomy, who used similar methods. Together they transformed the hospital from an auxiliary to an integral part of medical education. Moreover, the emphasis on science and research at Johns Hopkins symbolized a significant shift from the time when students "read" medicine and the professors were too busy with their practices to pay much attention to research. Finally, the extensive use of laboratories brought medical education in line with the developments of the bacteriological revolution. Perhaps the significance of the Johns Hopkins Medical School is most obvious from the fact that within two decades more than sixty American colleges had appointed three or more professors who held Hopkins degrees.[24] Thus, the innovative ideas demonstrated in Baltimore were disseminated throughout the nation, and men who had been infused with an appreciation for scientific research brought their enthusiasm to institutions that had always emphasized the practical rather than the scientific nature of medicine.

The Johns Hopkins experience demonstrated that a superior medical college *could* be developed in the United States as long as the school was not dependent upon student fees. Since the school was endowed and affiliated with a university, it was able to develop innovations that served to improve American medical education. Medical reformers of the past had recognized the need to make the schools truly independent, but little had been done in that direction until the Johns Hopkins experiment.[25]

Similarly, others had recognized the need for extensive clinical teaching, but little had been done to develop that to its logical conclusion, as was done in Baltimore.[26] Earlier some colleges had affiliated with hospitals, but the hospital work either was not required or it was not an integral part of the medical curriculum. The historian cannot but get the impression that the early developments in this area were primarily intended to enable the colleges to *advertise* that they had ample hospital beds for clinical study, but when the students enrolled, they might have found that the "hospital" consisted of three beds in an attic or that its use consisted of professors sweeping through in a hurried clinical lecture.

By the turn of the century, it came to be generally recognized that hospital training was an integral part of medical education. In 1900 the *Journal of the American Medical Association* declared: "Indeed, to a large extent, the hospital, with its wards, its out-patient department, its operating-rooms, its dead-house, and its laboratories, *is the medical school*." [27] To a large extent, Johns Hopkins paved the way for this development.

The college also demonstrated the advantage of affiliation with a university. In 1888 William Henry Welch described the benefits of the German system, where medical colleges were departments within prestigious universities. Welch noted that a close relationship with a university maintained the proper balance between the "purely technical training" and the more practical aspects of medical science. The university would provide the laboratories needed for premedical training, while the medical school could coordinate the practical training so necessary for the successful practice of medicine. Affiliation with a well-equipped university would encourage medical research by making available the best of laboratory facilities and attracting professors with an interest in science. Finally, and most important considering the state of medical education of the time, a medical department of a university would be more likely to receive an endowment than would a proprietary medical college. Thus, affiliation with a university could help reduce the dependence upon student fees, which would enable the college to improve standards without fear of the economic consequences. [28]

Once again, the European influence is apparent. The bacteriological revolution resulted in an emphasis on medical science rather than the art of medicine; to a large extent, the revolution was centered in Germany. Moreover, as medical knowledge increased as a result of developments in physiology and other basic sciences, it made the general practitioner an anachronism. There was a definite trend toward specialization, a trend enabling physicians to become experts in one branch of medical science. And many of the leading specialists in the world were teachers in German universities. As a result, from 1870 to 1914, many of the most ambitious young American physicians did postgraduate work in Germany. Just as Edinburgh had replaced Leyden as the leading medical center of the eighteenth century and Paris had taken that position in the early nineteenth century, Germany became the medical capital of the world in the late nineteenth century.[29]

When the American physicians returned to the United States, they began "to add their voices to those already working for a complete overhaul of American medical education." They had taken advantage of real postgraduate study, and they noted that the German medical schools were branches of universities, with full-time professors and well-equipped laboratories. By comparison, American schools were clearly deficient. It seemed obvious that in order to produce modern, scientifically oriented physicians, the German example had to be followed. Although the German universities had no rigid curriculum, students were encouraged to take the basic sciences, followed by pathology and pharmacology. Finally, they would conclude their courses with work in the clinical specialties. In order to advance to the clinical years, students had to pass examinations in the basic sciences. The German universities, in effect, had the graded curriculum that was absent in the United States. In addition, the German medical schools admitted only students who had a certain level of premedical training.[30]

Rather interestingly, while the drive to improve the quality of American medical education was receiving its impetus from the German experience, medical education in Germany seemed to be moving away from the American ideal. Early in the nineteenth century, the various German states had medical examining boards to ensure that unqualified physicians would not be able to practice medicine. In 1901, however, the state gave the right to license physicians back to the medical professors, apparently believing that the experts who taught at the universities were competent to judge their own students.[31] Yet it was a dangerous precedent, as evident from the American experience.

In any case, the movement was clear. The German influence was crucial. Johns Hopkins was based on the German model, and men who were trained in Germany staffed the new or reformed medical schools, including Harvard, Michigan, and Cornell. They followed the examples of their German professors, lecturing less and demonstrating more. They strove for higher entrance standards, a more flexible curriculum, an expansion of the basic sciences, and like the German system, they sought to affiliate with good universities.[32]

Notes

1. See above, pp. 67-69, 121-124, 130-131.
2. John H. Rauch, "Address on State Medicine," *JAMA* 6 (June 12, 1886): 645-652; James R. Parsons, Jr., "Preliminary Education, Professional Training and Practice in New York," *JAMA* 26 (June 13, 1896): 1149-1152. For a brief history of medical licensing, see Richard H. Shryock, *Medical Licensing in America* (Baltimore, 1967).
3. See above, p. 68.
4. *New York Medical Journal* 20 (1874): 64-72.
5. *New England Medical Gazette* 20 (July 1885): 323-329.
6. *American Homeopath* 10 (January 1884): 26.
7. Ibid. (March 1884): 86.
8. William Osler, "The License to Practice," *Transactions of the Medical and Chirurgical Faculty of the State of Maryland, 1889* (Baltimore, 1889), pp. 70-72.
9. *New York Medical Journal* 52 (July 12, 1890): 46.
10. Ibid. 55 (February 13, 1892): 182; (February 27, 1892): 240-241.
11. Ibid. 61 (February 16, 1895): 212-213.
12. *New York Times,* February 26, 1907.
13. *Medical Record* 71 (May 18, 1907): 820; *Hahnemannian Monthly* 41 (June 1907): 463-466; *JAMA* 49 (November 30, 1907): 1867.
14. See David L. Cowen, *Medicine and Health in New Jersey* (Princeton, 1964), pp. 74, 129-132; *Hahnemannian Monthly* 28 (March 1893): 198-200; and see, for example, *Homeopathic Recorder* 26 (August 1911): 337-339.
15. Parsons, "Preliminary Education," 1149-1152.
16. Samuel James Crowe, *Halsted of Johns Hopkins* (Springfield, Illinois, 1957), pp. 4-14.
17. Association of American Medical Colleges, *Proceedings, 1917,* p. 35.
18. Crowe, *Halsted,* pp. 4-14.
19. Richard H. Shryock, "The Influence of the Johns Hopkins University

on American Medical Education," *Journal of Medical Education* 31 (April 1956): 228-229.

20. James H. Cassedy, *Charles V. Chapin and the Public Health Movement* (Cambridge, Massachusetts, 1962), pp. 17-18.

21. Alan M. Chesney, *The Johns Hopkins Hospital and the Johns Hopkins University School of Medicine: A Chronicle* (Baltimore, 1943) 1: 85-93.

22. Ibid., 102-104; Shryock, "The Influence of the Johns Hopkins University," 230. See also Harvey Cushing, *Life of Sir William Osler* (Philadelphia and London, 1922), passim.

23. See Shryock, "The Influence of the Johns Hopkins University," 230.

24. An excellent description of the Johns Hopkins Hospital and College is given in Lewellys F. Barker, *Time and the Physician* (New York, 1942), pp. 36ff, 84ff.

25. See, for instance, the remarks of Frank Hastings Hamilton in the *New York Daily Tribune*, January 20, 1879.

26. Charles F. Withington, *The Relations of Hospitals to Medical Education* (Boston, 1886). For the history of another pioneering hospital, see Richard M. Doolen, "The Founding of the University of Michigan Hospital: An Innovation in Medical Education," *Journal of Medical Education* 39 (January 1964): 50-57.

27. *JAMA* 35 (August 25, 1900): 501. The italics are mine.

28. William Henry Welch, *Papers and Addresses* (Baltimore, 1920), 3: 26-40.

29. Thomas N. Bonner, *American Doctors and German Universities* (Lincoln, Nebraska, 1963), pp. 18-19.

30. Hans H. Simmer, "Principles and Problems of Medical Undergraduate Education in Germany during the Nineteenth and Early Twentieth Centuries," in C. D. O'Malley, ed., *The History of Medical Education* (Berkeley, Los Angeles, and London, 1970), pp. 182-186. See also Theodor Billroth, *The Medical Sciences in the German Universities* (New York, 1924), and Theodor Puschmann, *A History of Medical Education* (New York, 1966), pp. 584-598.

31. Simmer, "Principles and Problems of Medical Undergraduate Education in Germany," pp. 184-185.

32. Bonner, *American Doctors and German Universities*, pp. 57-63.

10
The Association
of American
Medical Colleges

Johns Hopkins University played a major role in bringing about a renewal of the effort to improve American medical education, and not simply by providing an example of the superior institution. Early in 1890 a series of meetings was held in Baltimore to discuss the need for nationwide reform, based on the ideals set by Johns Hopkins. Representatives of Maryland medical colleges gathered, and they decided that it would be self-destructive for all the colleges in one state to set high standards. As a result they called a convention of medical teachers to gather on May 21, 1890, prior to the American Medical Association's Nashville convention.[1]

Notice was sent to every allopathic medical institution, inviting each to send a delegate to a conference on "Medical Education in this Country and Measures for Its Improvement." The announcement included five items for discussion at the meeting, including consideration of a three-year program, with each term lasting at least six months, a graded curriculum, written and oral examinations, admission determined by examination, and laboratory instruction in chemistry, histology, and pathology. The letter was signed by two of Baltimore's leading physicians, Aaron Friedenwald and Eugene F. Cordell, who had been instructed to arrange the conference.[2]

Delegates of fifty-five of the ninety orthodox medical colleges in the country attended the meeting at Nashville. In their most significant decision, they established the National Association of Medical Colleges, an organization later called the Association of American Medical Colleges. When they began to discuss items on the agenda, there was a great deal of agreement. Delegates decided that in order to be members of the association, schools had to require three years of medical study for graduation, with the annual term not less than six months long. Moreover, every student had to pass oral and written examinations, and laboratory work had to be required in chemistry, histology, and pathology. Finally, the member institutions could no longer admit unqualified students; entrance examinations would be required, consisting of a two-hundred-word composition, translation of easy Latin prose, and tests in higher arithmetic and elementary physics. Graduates of recognized colleges of literature, science, or art, and normal schools, were exempted from this requirement.[3] Rather appropriately, N. S. Davis, who had been active in the cause of medical reform since back in the 1840s, was elected president of the association.

In 1891 the association was joined in the struggle for reform by the National Confederation of State Medical Examining and Licensing Boards, which voted to require a minimum of three years of medical training.[4] This type of dual effort was necessary; moral suasion had been unsuccessful in the past due to the absence of means of enforcing the decisions of either the AMA or the earlier American Association of Medical Colleges. When the reform was made a requirement for licensing, rather than dependent upon the goodwill of the various colleges, there was a greater chance of success.

For the first time, a nationwide attempt at reform was successful. By January 1893 less than 10 percent of the schools continued to have two-year courses. In fact, four institutions, Pennsylvania, Harvard, Michigan, and the Chicago Medical College, had four-year courses, and their enrollments had increased.[5] In 1894 the Illinois State Board of Health reported that in 1893, 96.3 percent of the schools required three or more years of study. This was a significant change; in 1880 only 26.8 percent of the colleges required that much work.[6]

The benefits offered by the better schools were becoming obvious; the results of the examining boards indicated that 25 percent of the graduates of inferior colleges were incapable of passing the required examinations, compared with 1.5 percent of the graduates of the better schools.[7] In addition, by 1892 twelve states required examination of all applicants before licensing.[8] This trend was obvious; eventually every state would require examination before licensure, making it likely that graduates of inferior schools would not be able to practice medicine in the United States.

In 1894 twenty-one of the seventy-one members of the Association of American Medical Colleges met in San Francisco and voted to extend the requirements to a four-year course of study to be effective for the graduating class of 1899. Those who attended that meeting understood that their actions would decrease membership in the association, but by then it was clear that the association was not crying alone in the wilderness—its actions were consistent with developments on the state level. The secretary of the association was instructed to cancel the registration of those institutions that "desired to withdraw their membership owing to the adoption of the four-years' curriculum."[9] The membership list did decrease—from around sixty-six in 1895 to fifty-four in 1897.[10] That was a great improvement over the situation in 1882 when more than half of the members of the old American Association of Medical Colleges withdrew in response to increased standards.[11]

By the middle of the 1890s, it was obvious that a great change had taken place in medical education, a change that coincided with the establishment of the association and the corresponding increased standards of medical licensure on the state level. Much more had to be done, but this was the most encouraging period in the history of the reform movement to that date.

The improvements, and the future needs, could be seen in the studies of Frederick H. Gerrish, an officer of the Maine State Board of Health. Back in 1887 Gerrish had set out to determine the situation among the colleges through what he referred to as his "detective work." He had an eight-year-old girl, "whose handwriting . . . gave ample evidence of the immaturity of the writer," apply to a number of medical schools. In each application, she "confessed her absolute ignorance of natural philosophy or some other study" required of all applicants at that time.[12]

The response from the colleges was shocking although not unexpected. About half of the schools "evinced a willingness to take the fee of the applicant, and promised to make a doctor of her in spite of her confessed inability to pass the examination prescribed in their prospectuses as necessary to gain admission to their halls." One school wrote: "Our examination is not difficult; no one has yet failed to pass." Another wrote: "The preliminary examinations are not difficult, and no deserving applicant is rejected on account of not being able to pass them. Call and see me when you are in the city, and I will fix it so you can enter."[13] According to Gerrish, half the colleges indicated an honest willingness to abide by the accepted standards of the day. The remainder, however, "fairly tumbled over each other in their indecent scramble to secure this prospective student, who frankly proclaimed his unfitness even according to their miserable standard."[14]

This survey took place after the old American Medical College Association had disbanded as a result of its inability to bring about reform and while the colleges were allowed to continue with their unprofessional competition. In 1891 and 1892 Gerrish set out to determine whether there had been any changes over the past six years, during which the new association had been established and while the process of medical licensure was being overhauled. He once again had letters sent to those colleges that had demonstrated a lack of standards in the earlier survey. The writer made certain to explain that he could "not undertake to acquaint himself with Latin and natural philosophy," which every college described in their announcements as prerequisites.[15]

Gerrish was able to report that *some* schools had obviously reformed. For instance, one New York school had replied in 1887: "The examination is not difficult. Reading, spelling, writing, arithmetic, and geography are the principal things touched upon. No one has as yet failed to pass them." In 1893 the same college informed the applicant: "The New York State law requires preliminary examinations in English branches, and the Faculty in addition requires Algebra, Geometry, and Latin. These examinations have to be passed without conditions before college work is begun!"[16] Other schools declared their willingness to admit the candidate, provided he pass the required examinations before graduation. A third group of colleges did not quite say so, but "craftily" implied that they were "willing to violate their regulations for the benefit of an avowed ignoramus."[17] Finally, some schools "come out flat-footed, and vociferously bid for anybody who can be induced to attend." A southern college declared: "The philosophy will give you no trouble whatever, and as for Latin, the amount required is very small. Do not let this stand in the way of coming to our college." Another institution, obviously in Chicago, informed the applicant: "We do not require Latin nor philosophy, but of course they are good studies and would help some. If you desire to study medicine we can give you first-class advantages and our offer is cheaper than any other first-class colleges in the country." In perhaps the most ironic touch, one southern school declared that although knowledge of Latin and natural philosophy were recommended, special consideration had always been given to "a practical man, who can wright [sic] a good letter (like yours)—and is well balanced and educated in all the practical walks of life."[18]

Even in the South, however, reform was on the way. As early as 1892 W. T. Briggs and G. C. Savage called a meeting to establish the Southern Medical College Association in the hope of upgrading medical education in the most backward section of the country. The South had once had some leading schools, in Kentucky and New Orleans, but the Civil War had wreaked havoc with them. During the war every southern college was forced to close. By the time they reopened they were at least twenty years behind the institutions of other sections. On November 16, 1892, representatives of eleven southern colleges gathered at Louisville, and they adopted two basic resolutions. First, they voted to improve the preliminary education of their students by agreeing to accept no one who did not possess the education required of second-grade public school teachers, namely completion of the first year of high school. Second, they agreed upon a common curriculum, with a three-year course, six months study per year, with dissection and hospital or clinical instruction. By 1898 the association had adopted a four-year graded curriculum, to become effective on January 1, 1899.[19]

The turn of the century saw a renewed effort by the American Medical Association in the area of medical education. At the AMA meeting in 1900, it was agreed that no society or organization would be allowed to have representation at future AMA conventions if it admitted anyone who received the MD degree in less than four years of graded instruction.[20] That was an important move for the AMA, which had hesitated to continue its drive to improve medical education following the failures of the past.[21]

In 1902 the president of the AMA, John A. Wyeth, appointed a five-man committee on education, which was chaired by Arthur Dean Bevan of Chicago. In 1903 the committee reported that since the AMA was in the process of being reorganized with a compact representative body, the house of delegates, it once again had the opportunity to become "the best national instrument to control and elevate medical education." The committee recommended that the association adopt an educational requirement for membership, based on preliminary education and a sufficient medical training. Moreover, it suggested that a permanent committee on medical education be established to secure the adoption of higher standards, to investigate the "character of work done by each medical school," and to inform the colleges of the AMA requirements.[22]

The report was referred to the trustees, who decided that reform of medical education might "be an obstacle in the way of the large plans for reorganization." Therefore the recommendations were tabled for one year to allow the reorganization to continue without interference from a possibly suicidal attempt to raise educational standards.[23]

At the 1904 convention, the committee on education again reported, and this time the delegates agreed to make the committee a permanent one that would prepare annual reports on the condition of American medical education and make suggestions on how to improve education and influence the colleges to accept higher standards. A conference was called for April 20, 1905, in Chicago in the hope that the AMA could gain the support of the state societies, the Association of American Medical Colleges, and the Southern Medical College Association in what would be the first coordinated assault on low standards in medical education.[24] Thus was born the AMA Council on Medical Education, which was to play a major role in the twentieth-century improvements in medical education.

By 1906 the council was evaluating the colleges and making recommendations that would ensure that future medical graduates would be fully qualified, both in terms of preliminary education and medical training. In 1906 the council presented its first report, which rated the colleges on the basis of the percentage of their students who failed to pass state board examinations. Basing their analysis on the 1904 reports published in the *Journal of the American Medical Association,* the council discovered that forty-seven colleges had fewer than 10 percent failures, twenty-seven schools had from 10 to 20 percent failures, and more than 20 percent of the students from the remaining thirty-eight institutions failed to pass the board examinations.[25]

The report declared that "there are five specially rotten spots that are responsible for most of the bad medical education." These were the states of Illinois, Kentucky, Maryland, Missouri, and Tennessee. In addition, the figures indicated that state examining boards were more lenient toward graduates of local colleges. More than 25 percent of the graduates of out-of-state colleges failed the examinations compared to only 9.2 percent of the local students.[26]

In the following year, 1907, the council reported the results of a three-year study of all the American colleges. The individual reports were read to the officials of the various institutions so they knew their rating and could make adjustments to ensure higher ratings in the next survey. The council openly implied that the results of the next survey would be publicized nationally, which might be catastrophic to some colleges. The public report in 1907 simply declared that of the 160 schools, "only about 50 percent are sufficiently equipped to teach modern medicine," 30 percent "are doing poor work," and 20 percent "are unworthy of recognition." The council noted that those states with inadequate medical license laws were becoming "dumping grounds" for graduates of the low-grade institutions who could not pass the medical boards in other states and who moved in large numbers to those states that did not require examination.[27]

When Arthur D. Bevan, the chairman of the council, made his 1907 report, he noted that when the council made its inspection, it

"found schools which are absolutely worthless, without any equipment for laboratory teaching, without any dispensaries, without any
hospital facilities, some which are no better equipped to teach
medicine than is a Turkish-bath establishment or a barbershop." In
addition, Bevan declared: "Many schools are conducted for the purpose of preparing a student to pass a state board examination and not
with the object of making him a competent practitioner."[28]

In 1906 the council began an attack on low standards in preliminary
education. It proposed that schools require not only a high school
education but at least one year of college. That was necessary in the
new scientific world of the twentieth century when physicians
needed a firm grounding in biology, chemistry, and physics. In 1909
Nathan P. Colwell, who was devoted to the cause of reform, prepared a report for the Council on Medical Education, which indicated that only fifteen schools required work beyond high school.[29]
Soon, however, it became obvious that there was a trend toward
increasing entrance requirements and that the recommendations of
the Association of American Medical Colleges and the AMA Council
on Medical Education were in fact being followed by the various
schools. Later in 1909 the council reported that seventeen schools
required two years of college, eleven others would require that
beginning in 1910, and twenty-two other institutions required one
year of college. A total of fifty schools, then, would soon require some
college work of all applicants.[30] This signaled a vast improvement in
the caliber of the American medical student. That is especially the
case when one considers that before 1900 Johns Hopkins was the only
school that required advanced work and before 1905 the only schools
that could claim such high standards were Johns Hopkins, Harvard,
Western Reserve, Rush, and the University of California.[31]

The drive to reform medical education was finally achieving some
success, success that was especially satisfying in view of past efforts
that invariably resulted in dismal failure. Through the work of Bevan
and Colwell, the AMA Council on Medical Education played a major
role in this early twentieth-century success. Bevan and Colwell
planned the council's surveys and investigations, and they issued
numerous reports on the quality of American medical education. It
was crucial for the colleges to be somewhat organized through the
Association of American Medical Colleges. This allowed for simul-

taneous rather than unilateral reform. Finally, the stringent laws in some states and the trend toward even stronger legislation in the future encouraged the schools to follow the recommendations of the association and the council. If the colleges refused to take action, they faced the very real possibility of being destroyed as a result of their inability to prepare their graduates for the state board examinations. The process of reform was finally well under way.

Notes

1. Dean F. Smiley, "History of the Association of American Medical Colleges, 1876-1956," *Journal of Medical Education* 32 (July 1957): 515; see also Dudley S. Reynolds, "The Present Status of the Medical Profession," *Journal of the American Medical Association* 20 (June 3, 1893): 618-619; William J. Means, "The History, Aims, and Objects of the Association of American Medical Colleges," *Proceedings, Association of American Medical Colleges 1919,* pp. 5ff.

2. Smiley, "History of the Association," 515; Association of American Medical Colleges, *Bulletin, 1892* (St. Paul, 1892).

3. *JAMA* 14 (June 7, 1890): 829-830.

4. Smiley, "History of the Association," 515-516.

5. *JAMA* 20 (January 7, 1893): 24.

6. Ibid. 22 (March 17, 1894): 393-394. See above, pp. 130-132.

7. Ibid. 20 (January 7, 1893): 24.

8. Association of American Medical Colleges, *Bulletin, 1892,* (St. Paul, 1892), p. 40.

9. Smiley, "History of the Association," 516; Association of American Medical Colleges, *Report of the Committee on Syllabus* (Chicago, 1895), p. 10.

10. Statistics gathered from Association of American Medical Colleges, *Bulletin, 1892* (St. Paul, 1892), p. 8, and its *Report of Committee on Syllabus,* p. 10.

11. See above, p. 139.

12. *New York Times,* September 8, 1887.

13. Ibid.

14. Frederick Henry Gerrish, "Report of the Committee on the Requirements for Preliminary Education in the Various Medical Colleges in the United States," *Bulletin of the American Academy of Medicine* 1 (February 1894): 435.

15. Ibid., 437.
16. Ibid.
17. Ibid., 437-438.
18. Ibid., 439.
19. G. C. Savage, "Medical Education in the South," *Bulletin of the American Academy of Medicine* 4 (October 1899): 358-375. See John Duffy, "A Note on Ante-Bellum Southern Nationalism and Medical Practice," *Journal of Southern History* 34 (May 1968): 266-276.
20. *JAMA* 34 (June 16, 1900): 1559.
21. See above, pp. 109-117.
22. AMA Council on Medical Education, *Report of the First Annual Conference, 1905* (Chicago, 1905), pp. 4-6.
23. Ibid., p. 7.
24. Ibid., pp. 7-8.
25. AMA Council on Medical Education, *Report of the Second Annual Conference, 1906* (Chicago, 1906), pp. 6-14.
26. Ibid.
27. AMA Council on Medical Education, "Medical Education in the United States," *Pamphlet Number 22* (Chicago, 1907); *New York Times,* July 12, 1907.
28. AMA Council on Medical Education, *Report of the Third Annual Conference, 1907* (Chicago, 1907), p. 10.
29. N. P. Colwell, "A Statement of Entrance Requirements," *Bulletin of the American Academy of Medicine* 10 (June 1909): 143-152. See also Association of American Medical Colleges, *Proceedings, 1908* (1908), p. 21.
30. *AMA Bulletin* 5 (September 15, 1909): 6-7.
31. Colwell, "A Statement of Entrance Requirements," 143-152.

11

The Flexner Report
And Its Aftermath

The work of the Council on Medical Education and the Association of American Medical Colleges was indeed crucial to the reform movement, yet it was insufficient, primarily because the two organizations were too closely related to the medical scene to be considered impartial observers. After all, medical societies had always fought the colleges for the control of licensing, and the association of colleges represented a group of schools that may have legitimately been accused of attempting to "control" medical education by destroying competition. Moreover, because the council and the association represented physicians and medical colleges, it was somewhat unethical for them to publicly condemn other physicians and colleges. Any public condemnation of the existing situation had to come from an outside agency that had no direct relationship with organized medicine, which could act from a moral stance. It could not be from an agency that might directly benefit from reform. That agency was to be the Carnegie Foundation for the Advancement of Teaching.

The work of the foundation in the area of medical education was closely connected with the work of the AMA Council on Medical Education, however. In 1907, for instance, Arthur Dean Bevan and Nathan P. Colwell invited Henry S. Pritchett, the president of the Carnegie Foundation, to inspect the results of the AMA survey of

American medical education. Undoubtedly Bevan and Colwell hoped that Pritchett could be encouraged to undertake an impartial survey which could be publicized and which could take the final step that the council could not—bring the conditions to the direct attention of the American people.[1] It should be noted that the desire to publicize the abuses was fully in line with the basic tenet of the Progressive reform movement of the day: "The truth shall make you free."

Pritchett was the perfect man to sponsor the survey; he was experienced both in science and education. Trained as an astronomer, he had taught at Washington University in St. Louis and had been director of the federal Coast and Geodetic Survey. In 1900 he became president of the Massachusetts Institute of Technology. Pritchett managed to convince Andrew Carnegie, the steel magnate, of the need for a philanthropic foundation to improve teaching; when the Carnegie Foundation was established, Pritchett became its president.[2]

Pritchett perceived the problems of medical education as educational ones rather than as simply medical ones. He obviously recognized that education for the professions had a history of its own; that medical and legal education, for instance, had struggled against many of the same problems. In order to place the history of medical education in this perspective, it is necessary to examine the major developments in the history of legal education.

During the colonial and early national periods, attorneys were trained through formal apprenticeship, with specific regulations determining the length of study. After having completed his apprenticeship, the prospective lawyer was admitted to practice by the courts. Then, in certain parts of the country, primarily in the northeast, judges began to permit "the bar"—the "judicially admitted practitioners"—to control entrance into the profession.[3] These developments correspond almost exactly with the situation in the medical profession during that period.

Then, as the impulse called Jacksonian democracy developed, state after state began to change the requirements for the practice of law. After all, control of the profession by the practicing lawyers was seen as a threat to the common man. Moreover, it seemed to be a self-serving monopoly that prevented competition. Since then, the power of admitting lawyers to practice has been a function of the bench rather than the bar. By 1860 only Ohio and North Carolina still required a definite period of study, and the laws in those states were not enforced. Formal apprenticeship gave way to a clerkship, and study did not even have to be under the direct supervision of an attorney. In addition, a stratified profession, with a distinction between practice before lower and upper courts, disappeared during Jackson's time.

During the period after 1870, the number of law schools proliferated—from fifteen schools in 1850, to thirty-one in 1870, sixty-one in 1890, and 124 in 1910. The schools developed at such a rapid pace to take advantage of the need for inexpensive, fast roads to legal education in the absence of the strict requirements of the past.[4]

The growth of corruption following the Civil War made reform of legal education inevitable. That was especially the case when it was easy to draw a relationship between low standards of education and the corrupt judges and politicians of the time. Rather significantly, in the midst of the exposure of the graft and corruption of the Tweed ring, the New York City Bar Association was established in 1870 in the hope of raising standards and eliminating some of the corruption. In 1878 the American Bar Association was organized, and a move developed to improve the situation by raising standards for admission to the profession. By 1890 nearly half of the states and territories required a specific period of study for admission to the bar.[5] These developments corresponded to the formation of the AMA and to the medical license laws of the postwar period.

As early as the 1860s, some law schools had moved toward reform. In 1863 Columbia instituted an optional third year for a master's degree, but this failed; only a handful of students wanted to prolong their education when they could easily practice, and profit, with the same training as the typical lawyers of the day. In 1872 Boston University was the first school to require a three-year course, and Harvard followed next. When those schools were able to remain in existence in spite of more stringent requirements, the three-year course became standard at the better law schools.[6] Law schools slowly and steadily improved, as did the medical schools of the day. By 1921 and 1922, for instance, there was only one one-year law school, and only fifteen law schools had two-year courses of study.[7]

When the Carnegie Foundation sponsored a survey of legal education, it took eight years to complete the research. When the report was published in 1921, it demonstrated that the system of legal education was in a state of chaos in spite of the improvements at some schools. Some colleges had no entrance requirements except the ability to pay the fees while others required college degrees for admission. In addition, the length of the course differed at various institutions. Indeed, in 1893, a committee of the American Bar Association reported that a course longer than two years was "impracticable for the greater number of schools." Yet the study of law had become more "complex and extensive with the multitude of decisions and statutes."[8] From this brief description of the history of legal education, it can be seen that the professions had gone through the same processes, in much the same way.

In 1908 Henry Pritchett recommended that the Carnegie Foundation undertake examinations of medical, legal, engineering, and theological education. The first step was to locate a qualified investigator to make a thorough analysis of medical education. Pritchett had read Abraham Flexner's *The American College,* a criticism of the elective and lecture system, and he asked Flexner if he would be willing to make a study of medical education. Flexner's immediate reaction was that Pritchett had confused him with his brother, Simon, who was director of the Rockefeller Institute for Medical Research.[9] When Pritchett explained that he wanted an analysis of American medical education from the perspective of educational theory and practice, Flexner consented to undertake the study.

Flexner, who knew very little about medical education, began by trying to familiarize himself with all phases of the problem. He delved into the literature, reading everything he could find on medical education. He studied Billroth's classic work on the European faculties as he tried to formulate standards by which to evaluate the American institutions. He read all the reports of the AMA Council on Medical Education, and he conferred with Bevan, Colwell, and George H. Simmons, the editor of the *Journal of the American Medical Association.* Flexner spent a great deal of time at Johns Hopkins, where he spoke with Welch, Halsted, Mall, and others who had developed the foremost American school. Ultimately he developed a view of the ideal college, "embodying," he said, "in a novel way, adapted to American conditions, the best features of medical education in England, France and Germany."[10]

Having developed a theoretical framework, Flexner set out to inspect the nation's medical colleges. He began at Tulane University in the winter of 1908, making a detailed analysis of the entire situation. He examined the entrance requirements to see whether they were sufficient and if they were enforced. He studied the size and training of the faculty, to determine if it was extensive enough and qualified to prepare students for the scientific practice of medicine. He made an analysis of the finances of the colleges in order to learn if the school was capable of providing the needed facilities. Then he inspected the laboratories. Finally he toured the hospital facilities to determine whether they were sufficient to provide ample clinical experience. Happily for Flexner, the college administrators totally misunderstood his mission. They believed that his survey would result in grants from the Carnegie Foundation, and they were "more than candid," happy to demonstrate inadequacies at their institutions.

The conditions he found were shocking, especially since there had been some improvement prior to his survey. For instance, when he asked the dean of one school whether the college had a physiological laboratory, the dean went upstairs "to get it," returning with a small sphygmograph, an instrument to measure the pulse. In an osteopathic college, Flexner found doors labeled "physiology," "anatomy," and so on, but when he had the janitor unlock the doors, he found no charts or apparatus in any of the "laboratories." Flexner's final report was brutally frank. He described Bowdoin College as "a disgraceful affair." The Birmingham Medical College was "a joint stock company, paying annual dividends of 6 percent." The California Medical College was "a disgrace to the state whose laws permit its existence."[11]

In order to fully appreciate Flexner's diligence, it is necessary to read the Flexner papers at the Library of Congress. In many colleges, he inspected the credentials of every student, and he then investigated to learn whether the students had really graduated from four-year high schools, as the colleges required. In a great many cases he found that the previous reforms in many colleges had been a sham, with students having "graduated" from two- or three-year high schools, and, in scattered cases, having "graduated" from "high schools" that had never existed.[12]

Flexner tracked down the records of students who had transferred from one medical college to another. In many cases he discovered that schools were giving advanced credit to transfer students who had failed their courses elsewhere. Schools that were chronic violators included the Atlanta College of Physicians and Surgeons, Baltimore College of Physicians and Surgeons, Chicago's College of Physicians and Surgeons, and the University of Maryland. A great many other institutions, however, gave advanced credit to undeserving students but not to the extent practiced by the chronic offenders.[13] In addition, Flexner found that a great many inadequately prepared students managed to enter the better schools "through the back door" by first enrolling at low-standard institutions and then transferring to schools with higher entrance requirements.

Not only did the Flexner report describe the programs and facilities of every college, but it made specific proposals for the development of a national system of medical education. Flexner analyzed population growth, projected the future need for medical care, and evaluated the various schools in terms of physical and financial ability to provide a modern medical education. On the basis of these factors, he recommended an overhaul of the entire system by reducing the number of colleges from 155 down to thirty-one regional institutions. In order to provide adequate preclinical laboratory facilities and an atmosphere conducive to scientific research, each medical school would be a department of a large university. In addition, the colleges would be situated in large cities, "where the problem of procuring clinical material . . . practically solves itself." For instance, New England would have two four-year medical colleges, Harvard and Yale. Dartmouth and the University of Vermont would be two-year institutions, with their students transferring to either Harvard or Yale for the clinical years of their education. In Flexner's plan, twenty states would be left without any medical schools because of insufficient demand for medical care, a lack of adequate universities, and an inability to financially support the truly modern institution.[14]

When the Carnegie Foundation published the report, the press completed Flexner's work. Newspapers from coast to coast, with few exceptions, accepted his findings as the truth. Editors demanded improvements in the local colleges. Professors at some schools attacked Flexner for being unfair, and others tried to explain that lack of funds had prevented their colleges from improving in the past. The Flexner report in effect was an obituary for a great many medical colleges.[15] Within a few years almost half of the colleges had disappeared; some were driven out of business by the adverse publicity and others merged with neighboring institutions.

The Flexner report demonstrated that the "commercial" schools, those operated to benefit the professors and trustees, were totally inadequate. Interestingly, Flexner's own evidence indicated that most of the professors did not directly benefit financially; they seemed to have been working for love of teaching and a sincere desire to advance American medicine.[16]

Possibly due to that sincerity, some officials defended themselves against what they considered to be Flexner's unwarranted attack. They insisted that the medical profession should not be restricted to those wealthy enough to have received the advanced education required for admission to the better schools. They declared that the "poor schools . . . existed for the poor boy." Some professors admitted that their facilities were inadequate, that their standards were low, and that their students were unprepared. They noted, however, that "every now and then in the army of the unfit" appears "a genius who eventually becomes a great physician or a great researcher." If not for these institutions, the argument continued, the world would lose the benefit of the genius who, through no fault of his own, had never had the opportunity to obtain a classical education.[17]

An editorial in *American Medicine* used Flexner's brother, Simon, as an example of the need for the "low standard" schools. Simon Flexner had graduated from the University of Louisville, and the editor declared that if such an institution produced one such man in a decade, "that school has justified its existence." That example, however, was a questionable one; Flexner did not receive his training at Louisville. In fact, he was there before that college had laboratories in either bacteriology or pathology. After his graduation he spent ten years at Johns Hopkins where he received his scientific training.[18]

Other defenders of the status quo insisted that low-standard medical schools were needed to provide physicians for rural America.
Men who had studied in the city and who had practiced at the urban
hospitals would not return to the country. Moreover, the cost of
obtaining a medical education in the city was far greater than in
country institutions. This meant that graduates of urban colleges had
larger investments in their educations, and they would remain in the
city where the practice of medicine was more lucrative. Because it
was difficult for someone who lived in the country to obtain a good
preliminary education, the rural schools could not establish restrictive entrance requirements or maintain high standards. Finally, it
was argued that as a result of all these factors, the demise of the
low-standard schools would inevitably lead to a scarcity of physicians
in small-town and rural America. Thus, "the inhabitants of a small
village or the resident on an isolated farm must accept this poor
medical attendance or none at all."[19]

An example of this type of argument is found in a letter defending
the work of the Chattanooga Medical College. The writer declared
that Chattanooga and other similar schools prepared "worthy,
ambitious men" who had risen "above their surroundings to become
family doctors to the farmers of the South, and to the smaller towns of
the mining districts." According to the argument, although the
requirements of these colleges were not as high as those of Harvard
or Johns Hopkins, their students were given a practical rather than a
scientific education; they were being trained to be family physicians
and not specialists. The closing of these second-rate institutions,
then, would result in a shortage of general practitioners.[20]

Professors at a number of schools made specific complaints about
Flexner's treatment of their institutions. President Frederick W.
Hamilton of Tufts University insisted that Flexner's report was too
harsh on the Tufts Medical School. In his reply, Flexner demonstrated that his report was correct, using as evidence Frederick C.
Waite's earlier investigation for the Association of American Medical
Colleges. Flexner agreed with Hamilton's assertion that "there is no
question whatsoever that Tufts College more than meets the requirements of the Association of American Medical Colleges." He
declared, however, that those "requirements are extremely low."

When Hamilton questioned Flexner's lack of medical credentials, Flexner noted, quite correctly, that medical education had suffered greatly by "being left entirely in the hands of medical men."[21]

In retrospect, some of the arguments the professors used were quite understandable. Flexner, for instance, heard from a number of individuals that because the colleges depended upon student fees, it was virtually impossible for a faculty to initiate reform. The Flexner report in effect condemned colleges for having low standards, while in many instances those standards were low of necessity rather than choice. A. W. Harris, the president of Northwestern University, complained that Flexner had emphasized the low admission requirements at Northwestern, yet when the school had required one year of college for admission in the session of 1907-1908, the size of the freshman class had decreased from 131 to 66.[22] Flexner's analysis of the American medical colleges was based upon standards that could be kept only by a handful of schools whose endowments could support the laboratories and clinical facilities required for modern medical training. In effect, then, Flexner was blaming the other colleges for their failure to do something that was virtually impossible—to reform without endowments, adequate clinical material, and so forth.[23] A major question that had to be answered in due time was what the schools could do "if neither the state nor private philanthropy" would endow them sufficiently to be completely independent of all financial considerations.[24]

The Flexner report made no note of the inherent differences among the schools in various sections of the country. If it was difficult for many northern schools to improve their standards, it was almost impossible for southern and rural schools to do so. The lack of adequate public education in the South prevented the application of a nationwide set of requirements. Further, the low level of compensation in the South and in rural America resulted in a need for a different type of practitioner. The demand was for a "cheap" doctor, quickly trained. It was ridiculous for a young man in the South to devote years to preparation in college and medical school, only to become a poorly compensated rural practitioner. It was unrealistic for southern institutions to be judged by standards relevant to Harvard, Johns Hopkins, and Pennsylvania.[25]

In addition, Flexner did not really consider the long-term effects of specialization nor did he consider future advances in medicine and how they might effect medical practice and education. Finally, the desire to limit the number of medical schools and the increase in standards and requirements took place in an atmosphere where there was a desire to impose ethnic and religious quotas in American society. During that time there was an attempt, eventually successful, to limit immigration, and many of the economically poor students were immigrants, or children of immigrants, and through no fault of their own their educational backgrounds had been limited. Thus, the increase in standards and requirements was indirectly aimed at that group.

The effect of the Flexner report and the continuing work of the AMA and the Association of Colleges was a drastic reduction in the number of medical schools and a vast improvement in the quality of medical education. But when the population explosion developed after World War II, there was a shortage of trained physicians to meet the nation's growing needs. This cannot be blamed on Flexner himself, as his projections of population figures could not foretell the future effects of the great depression and World War II on family size and fertility rates.

In balance, the Flexner report did lead to an improvement in the quality of medical care, although at the same time, in trying to develop a national system of medical education, it did not consider local factors. In addition, the report blamed the existing situation on the professors, who were virtually helpless when one considers the fact that reform from within the system was suicidal to the colleges. The problem, however, was that in order to improve the quality of education, Flexner had to use some model, and that inevitably was Johns Hopkins. By comparison, every medical school in the country failed in its attempt to provide modern medical training.

Flexner's role in improving medical education did not cease with the publication of his report for the Carnegie Foundation. He had made valuable contacts among the great philanthropists of his time, and he used his influence to secure grants to restructure some of the more promising medical schools. For instance, when Milton Winternitz became dean of the Yale University Medical School, he applied for funds to the General Education Board, John D. Rockefeller's charitable foundation. Flexner, the executive secretary, went to New

Haven where he surveyed the facilities and discussed the problems with the college president and others in the area. Then he informed Yale that if it could raise $500,000 locally, the General Education Board would match that sum. With proper planning, Yale was to be transformed into a great medical institution.[26]

Events at the University of Chicago were similar. As a result of an analysis of the entire situation, Flexner decided that more than $5 million was needed to turn the Rush Medical College into a modern medical school. He convinced Julius Rosenwald, the head of Sears, Roebuck, to donate $500,000, and Flexner was able to commit the General Education Board and the Rockefeller Foundation to grants totaling $2 million. A local campaign was initiated to raise the remaining funds. The citizens of Chicago subscribed what they could, and when the drive was nearing its goal, Max Epstein and Albert Lasker donated the remainder. At that point, enough had been raised to place the University of Chicago Medical College into the same category as Johns Hopkins, Harvard, and Pennsylvania.[27]

Washington University in St. Louis was another institution transformed through the work and influence of Abraham Flexner. His preliminary report had indicated that the school was "a little better than the worst . . . but absolutely inadequate in every essential respect." Robert S. Brookings, who had been pouring $80,000 a year into the college, could hardly believe Flexner's analysis. Brookings rushed to New York City to confer with Flexner and Pritchett. It was decided that Flexner would reinspect the school and that he would give Brookings a tour of his own institution. They went to the dean's office where Flexner used the college records to show Brookings that the school accepted inadequately prepared students. Then they toured the facilities, and Flexner demonstrated the inadequacy of the laboratories. By the end of the inspection, Flexner had convinced Brookings that the best course would be to "abolish the school" and effect a total reorganization, with an improved faculty, better facilities, and higher standards. Flexner urged Brookings to take the lead in raising an endowment necessary to "repeat in St. Louis what President Gilman accomplished in Baltimore." As a result, Washington University was to take the first steps toward that goal.[28]

Flexner even played a role in improving Johns Hopkins, which had been the model of perfection for his 1910 report. When Flexner went to Europe to study medical education in other lands, he met Franklin P. Mall, Johns Hopkins professor of anatomy; together they toured the institutions of the Old World. Mall, a firm advocate of full-time clinical teaching, apparently convinced Flexner of the benefits of the European system of medical education. When Flexner returned to the United States, he was asked by Frederick T. Gates, the chairman of the General Education Board, what he would do if he were given a million dollars to "make a start in the work of reorganizing medical education." Flexner's reply was simple—he would give it to Dr. Welch. Considering how much Welch had done at Johns Hopkins with a $400,000 endowment, Flexner could hardly imagine what could be done with an additional million. Gates then asked Flexner to prepare a report on the financial needs of Johns Hopkins.[29]

At a dinner at the Maryland Club, Flexner asked Welch, Mall, and Halsted what they would do if they were given a million dollars. Mall declared that he would use it to provide adequate salaries for the clinical staff. They had done wonders as part-time medical educators, he said, and "they could do still better with full-time."[30] After that meeting, Flexner recommended that the General Education Board give more than a million dollars to the school to put the medical, surgical, pediatric, and obstetric staff on a full-time basis.

William Osler, who had resigned in 1904 to return to England, was outraged when he learned of the proposal. He was apparently upset at the implication that he and his clinical colleagues had grown rich on their private practices, while the scientific faculty had labored under the burden of comparatively inadequate salaries. He was also convinced that practicing physicians made the best clinical teachers. Osler fired broadside after broadside at the plan, and Welch hesitated more than two years before finally accepting the grant in 1913. That enabled William Halsted, Theodore Janeway, and John Howland to assume full-time chairs in surgery, medicine, and pediatrics. For the first time, medical education and medical research had become full-time occupations for every member of the executive faculty of an American institution.[31]

The medical profession was divided by that utopian innovation. Although it was an admirable idea to have full-time clinical professors, there were a number of problems with the proposal. First, in order to persuade nationally recognized clinicians to assume full-time duties in the colleges, it was necessary to provide them with much higher salaries than those given to the scientific faculty. To some, this was outrageous. The AMA Council on Medical Education pointed out that "the sweating of the scientific men who have devoted their lives to teaching and research on miserable salaries is notorious" and that they "are often as underpaid comparatively as the workers in a sweat shop." The development of full-time clinical chairs also deprived the colleges of some exceptional teachers who were not willing to abandon their lucrative private practices. The prime example was Llewellys Barker of Johns Hopkins, who decided to step aside in favor of Theodore Janeway, who *was* willing to become a full-time teacher and researcher.[32]

In 1914 the AMA appointed a ten-man committee to study the need for a "thorough reorganization of clinical teaching." The committee consisted of some of the leading men in the profession, including Victor C. Vaughan of the University of Michigan, Frank Billings of the Rush Medical College, Harvey Cushing of Harvard, George Dock of Washington University, and William J. Mayo of Rochester, Minnesota. The committee report supported full-time clinical teaching on the grounds that it would prevent busy practitioners from neglecting their teaching duties in favor of the more lucrative private practice. Although the debate over full-time clinical staff continued well into the 1920s, it was the start of a significant movement to make medical education more of a full-time occupation than it had ever been before.[33]

Meanwhile the Council on Medical Education continued with its drive to eliminate the inferior medical colleges. In 1913, after an exhaustive evaluation and inspection of every school, the council announced its ratings. Twenty-four schools were considered to be class A+, those providing a high level of medical training. Thirty-seven colleges rated class A, acceptable but "lacking in certain respects." Another twenty-four colleges were placed in class B, which indicated that they needed general improvements to become acceptable. Finally, twenty-eight medical schools were relegated to class C, which indicated that they were not only providing an inferior medical education but that they required a thorough reorganization in order to become acceptable.[34]

By 1913 medical examining boards in twenty-four states refused to license graduates of class C schools. That significant development forced the class C schools to either make the necessary reorganization, which often was financially impossible, or to close their doors. With the state boards refusing to license the graduates, schools in that category could not attract students. Since in almost every case these schools depended upon student fees for financial support, that meant that the colleges really had no choice; they would disappear from the scene.[35]

As a result of the combined efforts of the Council on Medical Education, the Association of American Medical Colleges, and the various state medical examining boards, there was a general improvement of requirements and standards in the colleges. After January 1, 1914, seventy-seven schools required at least one year of college work, a necessary change due to the fact that many state boards refused to examine graduates of schools that did not meet that generally accepted admission requirement. In 1914 N. P. Colwell, who had been so active in the Council on Medical Education, reported on the year's progress. He noted that 85 percent of the colleges required one year of college work for admission, and twenty-five state boards required that for licensing. In addition, thirty-one state boards refused to recognize class C institutions. Finally, Colwell noted that more than 75 percent of the medical graduates were becoming hospital interns and that five colleges required their graduates to serve a fifth hospital year.[36]

In 1915 when the Council on Medical Education developed its ratings, it decided to eliminate class A+; many of the schools formerly rated in class A had made substantial improvements. Also, the AMA House of Delegates directed the council not to rate as class A any school that did not require a premedical college year, and the delegates also instructed the council not to rate higher than class C "any school that is owned and conducted as a private venture."[37]

An interesting and revealing encounter occurred at the 1915 meeting of the Association of American Medical Colleges. Henry S. Pritchett delivered a paper in which he complained that the AMA ratings were far too lenient. He pointed out that the highest class included "not only the strong medical schools with large endowments, complete clinical facilities and research departments," schools like Harvard, Johns Hopkins, Columbia, Cornell, and

Washington University, but it also included "institutions like Vanderbilt, Tulane, and Texas, whose standards and facilities are of an
entirely different order." In addition, Pritchett noted that the rating
"has been stretched to include schools of the type of the College of
Medicine at Omaha, and the Starling-Ohio School at Columbus."
Pritchett angrily declared that to group these with Harvard, Johns
Hopkins, and Washington University "is to wipe out real distinction."[38]

N. P. Colwell responded to the charges by admitting that the
ratings of the Council on Medical Education had been lenient. He
explained that the council had been trying to advance at a reasonable
pace. If the council insisted on too rapid reform, the result would be
the destruction of promising schools. On the other hand, if the
council favored a slow advance, the inadequate schools would be able
to continue to produce inferior physicians.[39]

In 1915 the slow but steady reform was to be given a boost by the
organization of the National Board of Medical Examiners. William L.
Rodman of Philadelphia recognized that a major problem was that
there was a wide variety of standards and requirements. What was
happening was that inferior schools recommended that their students move to states where the medical licensing boards were
lenient. On May 5, 1915, the national board was established, including some of the most prestigious members of the profession: Rodman, W. C. Braisted, the surgeon-general of the navy, W. C. Gorgas
of the United States Army, Isadore Dyer of New Orleans, Victor C.
Vaughan of the University of Michigan, and Austin Flint, Jr., of New
York City. At its meeting of November 29, the board adopted the
standards of the Council on Medical Education. Its ultimate goal was
to establish a national examination that would supersede the state
licensing boards and that would provide nationwide standards in
terms of admission requirements, educational standards, and college
training. Soon, the National Board of Medical Examiners was highly
considered in all medical circles, and its standards encouraged state
boards to raise their own expectations.[40]

In 1924 Abraham Flexner evaluated the changes that had taken
place in American medical education. He noted that since 1910
almost half of the colleges had disappeared. "The weak schools in all
sections of the country, particularly in the South and West, where

they were most abundant, have been almost wholly eliminated." There had been a general improvement of equipment and facilities in the existing medical schools. Everywhere laboratory subjects were taught by full-time, specially trained professors. Flexner was happy to report that there had been "a great reform" in the medical curriculum. The two- or three-year nongraded medical courses of the past had been replaced by a four-year graded curriculum, separating the preclinical from the clinical subjects.[41]

Flexner noted that a lot of work was yet to be done. Clinical instruction was still inadequate. "The busy practicing physician is still in most schools the teacher of the clinical subjects." In addition, clinical instruction was often "given in hospitals neither organized, equipped nor primarily meant for educational use." "In general," he continued, "the vast educational potentialities of city and state hospitals are either wasted or very ineffectively utilized." Flexner recognized that perfection had not been achieved through the improved educational standards of the early twentieth century. Every college required four years of high school and two years of college training, but "the high school situation in America is utterly chaotic and the college situation hardly less so." "It means one thing to be a graduate of the Boston Latin School and an entirely different thing to be the graduate of a four-year rural high school."[42]

A great deal of work was still to be done, but it would be easier to achieve reform in the future than it had been in the past. The existence of the Council on Medical Education and the Association of American Medical Colleges was no longer questioned. These national agencies were able to evaluate the contemporary situation, make recommendations for improvements and alterations, and when necessary, raise standards; colleges would be forced to comply or be threatened with loss of accreditation. Changes in the future were to alter a modern system rather than to transform an obsolete one, as had been the case with the reform movements of the period from 1890 to 1920.[43] The credit for the elimination of an archaic system and the development of a modern one must be given to these two organizations and to such individuals as N. S. Davis, N. P. Colwell, Arthur Dean Bevan, and Abraham Flexner, each of whom left his imprint on the drive to advance American medical education into the twentieth century.

Notes

1. Abraham Flexner, *Henry S. Pritchett: A Biography* (New York, 1943), p. 108. For a brief analysis of the role of Flexner, see Robert P. Hudson, "Abraham Flexner in Perspective," *Bulletin of the History of Medicine* 46 (November-December 1972): 545-561.

2. Flexner, *Henry S. Pritchett*, passim; see also Abraham Flexner, *Abraham Flexner: An Autobiography* (New York, 1960), pp. 70-71.

3. Alfred Z. Reed, *Training for the Public Profession of the Law* (New York, 1921), p. 36. See also Charles Warren, *History of the American Bar* (1913).

4. Reed, *Training for the Public Profession*, pp. 38-43, 86-87, 193.

5. Ibid., pp. 90-91.

6. Ibid., pp. 176-180.

7. Ibid., pp. 180-193.

8. Reed's study *was* the Carnegie Foundation survey of legal education. See also American Bar Association, *Report on Legal Education* (Washington, D.C., 1893), pp. 13-14. For a brief historical survey of other professions, see Lloyd E. Blauch, ed., *Education for the Professions* (Washington, D.C., 1955).

9. Flexner, *Pritchett*, p. 108.

10. Flexner, *Autobiography*, pp. 74-78; Flexner, *Pritchett*, p. 110.

11. Abraham Flexner, *Medical Education in the United States and Canada* (New York, 1910), passim; Flexner, *Autobiography*, pp. 80ff.

12. For examples, see Flexner to S. E. Weber, New York, August 17, 1909, and J. J. Doster to Flexner, June 12, 1909, Flexner Papers, Library of Congress.

13. Determined from Flexner papers.

14. Flexner, *Medical Education in the United States and Canada*, pp. 143ff.

15. Flexner, *Pritchett*, p. 113.

16. "Note on Weak Medical Schools," typescript, Flexner Papers, box 21.

17. Ibid.

18. Ibid.

19. Henry S. Pritchett, "The Obligations of the University to Medical Education," *AMA Bulletin* 5 (January 15, 1910): 291-292.

20. Copy in Flexner Papers, Chattanooga file.

21. See Hamilton to Pritchett, Boston, February 19, 1910, Flexner to Hamilton, New York, March 15, 1910, Flexner Papers, Tufts file. For similar material from other schools, see files of Lincoln Medical College, Denver-Gross Medical College, St. Louis College of Physicians and Surgeons, and the University of North Carolina.

22. See files of Northwestern University and University of Nashville, Flexner Papers.

23. See James J. Walsh to Henry S. Pritchett, New York, March 28, 1910, Fordham University files, and J. W. Holland to Flexner, Philadelphia, January 5, 1909, Flexner Papers, Jefferson Medical College file.

24. *Chicago Record-Herald,* June 7, 1910.

25. See Edwin B. Craighead, "Medical Education in the South," *AMA Bulletin* 7 (March 15, 1912): 230; and Flexner Papers, Chattanooga Medical College file.

26. Flexner, *Autobiography,* pp. 161ff.

27. Ibid., pp. 167-174; see also pp. 196ff. and Edward Mims, *Chancellor Kirkland of Vanderbilt* (Nashville, 1940), pp. 213ff.

28. See Joseph Aub and Ruth Hapgood, *Pioneer in Modern Medicine,* pp. 68-70, 110; Donna Bingham Munger, "Robert Brookings and the Flexner Report," *Journal of the History of Medicine* 23 (October 1968): 356-371.

29. Lewellys Barker, *Time and the Physician* (New York, 1942), pp. 188-195; Donald Fleming, "The Full-Time Controversy," *Journal of Medical Education* 30 (July 1955): 398-406.

30. Fleming, "The Full-Time Controversy."

31. The story is well told in Fleming's article.

32. AMA Council on Medical Education, *Report to the House of Delegates, 1914* (Chicago, 1914), p. 17; see Barker, *Time and the Physician,* pp. 193-195.

33. *AMA Bulletin* 10 (March 15, 1915): 244-268; see also the public debates in *New York Times,* October 27, 30, 31, November 6, 1921.

34. AMA, *Laws and Board Rulings Regulating the Practice of Medicine in the United States and Elsewhere,* 20th ed., rev. (Chicago, 1913), pp. 175ff.

35. AMA Council on Medical Education, *Report to the House of Delegates, 1913* (Chicago, 1913), pp. 14-15.

36. AMA Council on Medical Education, *Classified List of Medical Colleges in the United States, 1913* (Chicago, 1913), p. 16; N. P. Colwell, "Progress of the Year in Medical Education," *Report of the U.S. Commissioner of Education, 1914,* 1: 191, 197, 203, 216. The five colleges were Minnesota, Northwestern, Rush, Stanford, and the University of Vermont.

37. *AMA Bulletin* 10 (March 15, 1915): 227-230.

38. Henry S. Pritchett, "The Classification of Medical Schools," Association of American Medical Colleges, *Proceedings, 1915* (1915), p. 15.

39. Ibid., p. 24.

40. National Board of Medical Examiners, *Quarter of a Century of Progress* (Philadelphia, 1940), pp. 5ff.; J. S. Rodman, "Impressions on Medical Teaching Gained from Ten Years' Experience with National Board Examina-

tions," in Association of American Medical Colleges, *Proceedings, 1925* (1925), pp. 70ff. See also Nathan A. Womack, "The Evolution of the National Board of Medical Examiners," *JAMA* 192 (June 7, 1965): 817-823.

41. Abraham Flexner, "Medical Education, 1909-1924," *JAMA* 82 (March 15, 1924): 834-835.

42. Ibid., 834-837.

43. For modern trends, see Saul Jarcho, "Medical Education in the United States, 1910-1956," *Journal of the Mt. Sinai Hospital* 26 (1959): 339-385. See also Lamar Soutter, "Medical Education and the University, 1901-1968," *New England Journal of Medicine* 279 (August 8, 1968): 294-299; and C. Sidney Burwell, "Medicine as a Social Instrument: Medical Education in the Twentieth Century," *New England Journal of Medicine* 244 (May 3, 1951): 673-684.

Bibliography

Primary Sources

Private papers and manuscripts

John Shaw Billings Papers. National Library of Medicine, Bethesda, Maryland.

C. M. Bull Papers. Burton Historical Collection, Detroit Public Library.

Jonathan Edwards Papers. Boston Public Library.

Feamster Family Papers. Library of Congress, Washington, D.C. This collection includes an interesting diary, that of Charles William Cary, a young medical student.

Abraham Flexner Papers. Library of Congress, Washington, D.C.

John W. Francis Papers. Special Manuscript Collection, College of Physicians and Surgeons, Columbia University, New York City.

William Lloyd Garrison Papers. Boston Public Library.

Hamilton County Medical Club. Minutes. National Library of Medicine, Bethesda, Maryland.

Harvard Medical Faculty. Minutes, 1827-1841. Countway Library, Harvard University.

Benjamin Lincoln Papers. Countway Library, Harvard University.

John T. Mason Papers. Burton Historical Collection, Detroit Public Library.

Medical College of Ohio. Faculty Minutes, 1835, 1843. Archives of Medical History, University of Cincinnati Library.

William Prescott Papers. New York Public Library.

Thomas Ruston Papers. Library of Congress, Washington, D.C.

George C. Shattuck Papers. Massachusetts Historical Society, Boston, Massachusetts.

Sheldon Papers. Burton Historical Collection, Detroit Public Library.

Joseph Toner Collection. Library of Congress, Washington, D.C. This mas-

184   *Bibliography*

sive collection includes a volume of lecture notes by Alexander Clendinen from the lectures of Benjamin Rush in 1798.

Vermont Medical Society. Minutes. Wilbur Collection, Bailey Library, University of Vermont, Burlington, Vermont.

Wayne State University Archives. Detroit, Michigan. The archives include the alumni secretary's scrapbook number one, which includes numerous clippings on medicine in Michigan.

Official Records and Documents

American Bar Association. *Report on Legal Education.* Washington, D.C., 1893.

American Medical Association. *Transactions.* 1848-1872.

———. Council on Medical Education. *Classified List of Medical Colleges in the United States, 1913* (Chicago, 1913).

———. *Medical Education in the United States.* Chicago, 1907.

———. *Medical Schools of the United States, 1906.* Chicago, 1906.

———. *Report of the First Annual Conference of the Council on Medical Education, 1905.* Chicago, 1905.

———. *Report of the Second Annual Conference of the Council on Medical Education, 1906.* Chicago, 1906.

———. *Report of the Third Annual Conference of the Council on Medical Education, 1907.* Chicago, 1907.

———. *Report to the House of Delegates, 1913.* Chicago, 1913.

———. *Report to the House of Delegates, 1914.* Chicago, 1914.

American Medical College Association. *Proceedings.* 1878-1882.

Association of American Medical Colleges. *Bulletin.* 1892.

———. *Proceedings.* 1908, 1917.

———. *Report of the Committee on Syllabus.* Chicago, 1895.

Connecticut Medical Society. *Proceedings.* 1792-1834.

Proceedings of a Convention of Medical Delegates, Held at Northampton, June 20, 1827. Boston, 1827.

Illinois State Board of Health. *Annual Reports.* 1878-1882.

———. *Official Register of Physicians and Midwives.* Springfield, 1880.

Maine Medical Association. *Records of the Twelfth Annual Meetings, 1864-1865.* Portland, 1865.

Proceedings of the National Medical Conventions Held in New York, May, 1846, and in Philadelphia, May, 1847. Philadelphia, 1847.

Medical Society of New Jersey. *Transactions, 1766-1858.* Newark, 1875.

Ohio Medical Convention. *Journal of the Proceedings.* Cincinnati, 1835.

———. *Journal of the Proceedings.* Cincinnati, 1838.
———. *Proceedings of the Third Medical Convention.* Cleveland, 1839.
———. *Proceedings.* Columbus, 1847.
———. *Proceedings.* Columbus, 1848.

Newspapers

Boston Chronicle. 1768.
Boston Evening Post and General Advertiser. 1783.
Boston Gazette. 1766.
Chicago Record-Herald. 1910.
Cleveland Herald. 1833, 1842-1846.
Cleveland Leader. 1864.
Continental Journal and Weekly Advertiser (Boston). 1783.
Daily Advertiser (New York City). 1788.
Detroit Free Press. 1859.
Independent Reflector (New York City). 1753.
Maryland Journal and Baltimore Advertiser. 1785-1790.
Massachusetts Spy (Worcester). 1785.
National Gazette (Philadelphia). 1792.
New York Daily Tribune. 1875-1879.
New-York Mercury. 1765-1767.
New York Times. 1887-1921.
Pennsylvania Chronicle and Universal Advertiser. 1767.
Pennsylvania Gazette. 1762-1768.

Periodicals

AMA Bulletin. Vol. 5 (1909). Vol. 10 (1915).
American Homeopath. Vol. 10 (1884).
American Journal of the Medical Sciences. Vols. 20-23 (1837-1838).
American Medical Weekly. Vol. 4 (1876).
Atlanta Medical Journal. Vol. 4 (1859).
Boston Medical and Surgical Journal. Vol. 1 (1828). Vol. 106 (1883).
Bulletin of the American Academy of Medicine. Vol. 1 (1891).
Chicago Medical Journal and Examiner. Vol. 41 (1880).
Chicago Medical Review. Vol. 3 (1881).
Chicago Medical Times. Vol. 14 (1882).
Detroit Lancet. N.s. Vol. 4 (1880).

Hahnemannian Monthly. Vols. 28-41 (1893-1907).
Homeopathic Recorder. Vol. 26 (1911).
Journal of the American Medical Association. Vols. 14-49 (1890-1907).
Louisville Medical News. Vol. 1 (1876).
Medical and Surgical Reporter. Vol. 26 (1872).
Medical Communications of the Massachusetts Medical Society. Vol. 11
    (1874).
Medical News. Vol. 41 (1882).
Medical Record. Vols. 2-71 (1867-1907).
Nashville Journal of Medicine and Science. Vol. 19 (1860). N.s. Vol. 4 (1869).
New England Medical Gazette. Vol. 20 (1885).
New Orleans Medical and Surgical Journal. Vol. 23 (1870).
New York Medical Journal. Vols. 20-61 (1874-1895).
New York Medical Times. Vol. 17 (1889).
North American Review. Vol. 32 (1831).
North Carolina Medical Journal. Vol. 16 (1885).
St. Louis Medical and Surgical Journal. Vol. 12 (1854).
Stethoscope. Vol. 4 (1854).
United States Magazine, and Democratic Review. Vol. 22 (1848).

Books and Pamphlets

Abt, Isaac A. *Baby Doctor.* New York and London, 1944.
American Association of Medical Colleges. *History of Its Organization.*
    Detroit, 1877.
Barker, Lewellys F. *Time and the Physician.* New York, 1942.
Beck, T. Romeyn. *On the Utility of Country Medical Institutions.* Albany,
    1825.
Biddle, John B. *Materia Medica for the Use of Students.* 8th ed. Philadel-
    phia, 1878.
Bigelow, Jacob. *Nature in Disease.* Boston, 1854.
Boardman, Andrew. *Essay on the Means of Improving Medical Education
    and Elevating Medical Character.* Philadelphia, 1840.
Buchan, William. *Domestic Medicine, or the Family Physician.* Edinburgh,
    1769.
Buck, W. D. *Medical Education.* Manchester, New Hampshire, 1869.
Coates, Reynall. *Oration on the Defects in the Present System of Medical
    Instruction in the United States.* Philadelphia, 1835.
Cullen, William. *First Lines of the Practice of Physic.* New York, 1801.

Davis, N. S. *Address on the Progress of Medical Education.* Philadelphia, 1876.

————. *Contributions to the History of Medical Education and Medical Institutions in the United States of America. 1776-1876.* Washington, D.C., 1877.

————. *History of Medical Education and Institutions in the United States, from the First Settlement of the British Colonies to the Year 1850.* Chicago, 1851.

————. *History of the American Medical Association, from Its Organization up to January, 1855.* Philadelphia, 1855.

Drake, Daniel. *An Introductory Lecture, on the Means of Promoting the Intellectual Improvement of the Students and Physicians, of the Valley of the Mississippi, Delivered in the Medical Institute of Louisville, November 4, 1844.* Louisville, 1844.

————. *Practical Essays on Medical Education and the Medical Profession in the United States.* Cincinnati, 1832.

————. *Strictures on Some of the Defects and Infirmities of Intellectual and Moral Character, in Students of Medicine.* Louisville, 1847.

Ewell, James. *Planter's and Mariner's Medical Companion.* Philadelphia, 1807.

Flexner, Abraham. *Abraham Flexner: An Autobiography.* New York, 1960.

————. *Medical Education in the United States and Canada.* New York, 1910.

Godman, John D. *Monition to the Students of Medicine.* Philadelphia, 1825.

Gross, Samuel D. *Autobiography.* Philadelphia, 1887.

Hooker, Worthington. *Physician and Patient.* New York, 1849.

How, L. B. *Medical Education.* Manchester, New Hampshire, 1869.

Huston, Robert M. *Lecture Introductory to the Course on Materia Medica and General Therapeutics.* Philadelphia, 1852.

Jackson Samuel. *Medical Education.* Philadelphia, 1853.

Lincoln, Benjamin. *An Exposition of Certain Abuses Practiced by Some of the Medical Schools of New England and Particularly of the Agent-Sending System as Practiced by Theodore Woodward.* Burlington, Vermont, 1833.

————. *Hints on the Present State of Medical Education and the Influence of Medical Schools of New England.* Burlington, Vermont, 1833.

Lindsley, J. Berrien. *On Medical Colleges.* Nashville, 1858.

Manley, James. *Inaugural Address Delivered before the Medical Society of the State of New York.* New York, 1826.

Middleton, Peter. *A Medical Discourse, or an Historical Inquiry into the Ancient and Present State of Medicine.* New York, 1769.

Mitchell, J. K. *Lecture Introductory to the Course on the Practice of Medicine in the Jefferson Medical College.* Philadelphia, 1847.

Mitchell, Thomas D. *The Professor and the Pupil.* Philadelphia, 1862.

———. *The Study of Medicine.* Philadelphia, 1849.

Morgan, John. *A Discourse upon the Institution of Medical Schools in America.* Philadelphia, 1765.

Paine, Martyn. *A Defence of the Medical Profession of the United States.* 8th ed. New York, 1846.

Pepper, William. *Higher Medical Education.* Philadelphia, 1894.

Reese, David M. *The Humbugs of New York.* New York, 1838.

Rush, Benjamin. *Medical Inquiries and Observations.* 3d ed. Philadelphia, 1809.

Sewall, Thomas. *Lecture, Delivered at the Opening of the Medical Department of the Columbian College in the District of Columbia, March 30, 1825.* Washington, D.C., 1825.

Taylor, Othniel H. *Medical Reform and the Present System of Medical Instruction.* Camden, New Jersey, 1850.

Thomson, Samuel. *A Narrative of the Life and Medical Discoveries of Samuel Thomson; Containing an Account of His System of Practice, and the Manner of Curing Disease with Vegetable Medicine, upon a Plan Entirely New.* 5th ed. St. Clairsville, Michigan, 1829.

Toner, Joseph M. *Contributions to the Annals of Medical Progress and Medical Education in the United States Before and During the War of Independence.* Washington, D.C., 1874.

Welch, William Henry. *Papers and Addresses.* Baltimore, 1920.

White, James Clarke. *Sketches from My Life, 1833-1913.* Cambridge, Massachusetts, 1914.

Withington, Charles F. *The Relations of Hospitals to Medical Education.* Boston, 1886.

Wood, James D. *An Old Doctor of the New School.* Caldwell, Idaho, 1942.

Articles

Bigelow, Henry J. "Medical Education in America." *Medical Communications of the Massachusetts Medical Society* 11 (1874): 181-259.

Blachford, Thomas. "A Condensed Statement of What Has Been Attempted for the Advancement of Medical Education, by the Medical Conventions of 1846 and 1847, and by the A.M.A. Since Its Organization in

1847." *Transactions of the Medical Society of the State of New York* (1860): 120-138.

Cartwright, Samuel A. "Remarks on Statistical Medicine, Contrasting the Result of the Empirical with the Regular Practice of Physic, in Natchez." *Western Journal of Medicine and Surgery* 2 (July 1840): 1-21.

Chaille, Stanford E. "State Medicine and State Medical Societies." *Transactions of the American Medical Association* 30 (1879): 299-355.

―――. "The Medical Colleges, the Medical Profession, and the Public." *New Orleans Medical and Surgical Journal*, n.s. 1 (May 1874): 819-841.

Collins, A.H. "Principles and Progress of the Eclectic School of Medicine." *National Eclectic Medical Association Quarterly* 7 (March 1916): 267-276.

Colwell, N. P. "Medical Education." *Report of the United States Commissioner of Education, 1915* 1 (1915): 185-220.

―――. "Progress of the Year in Medical Education." *Report of the United States Commissioner of Education, 1914* 1 (1914): 191-216.

―――. "A Statement of Entrance Requirements." *Bulletin of the American Academy of Medicine* 10 (June 1909): 143-152.

Craighead, Edwin B. "Medical Education in the South." *AMA Bulletin* 7 (March 15, 1912): 219-231.

Crawford, S. P. "Medical Education." *Nashville Journal of Medicine and Surgery* 12 (February 1857): 101-105.

Davis, N. S. "The Earlier History of the Medical School." In Wilde, Arthur H. *Northwestern University: A History.* New York, 1905. Vol. 3: 298-308.

Delafield, Edward. "Sketch of the College of Physicians and Surgeons of the University of the State of New York." *New York Journal of Medicine* 3d ser. 2 (March 1857): 163-182.

Eve, Joseph A. "Medical Education." *Southern Medical and Surgical Journal* 1 (September 1836): 216-226.

Flexner, Abraham. "Medical Education, 1909-1924." *Journal of the American Medical Association* 82 (March 15, 1924): 833-838.

Gerrish, Frederick Henry. "Report of the Committee on the Requirements for Preliminary Education in the Various Medical Colleges in the United States." *Bulletin of the American Academy of Medicine* 1 (February 1894): 435-439.

Green, William W. "Private Preceptorship in the Study of Medicine." *Boston Medical and Surgical Journal* 105 (July 7, 1881): 25-29.

Holmes, Daniel. "An Essay on Medical Education." *Transactions of the Medical Association of Southern Central New York* (1854): 36-52.

Ingals, E. Fletcher. "A Review of the Progress of Medical Education in Chicago." *Chicago Medical Journal and Examiner* 42 (February 1881): 136-147.

Johnson, H. O. "The Regulations of Medical Practice by State Boards of Health." *Transactions of the American Medical Association* 30 (1879): 293-298.

King, Robert M. "Shall We Have a Higher Standard of Medical Education?" *St. Louis Clinical Record* 8 (March 1882): 341-348.

Lord, Asa D. "Medical Education." *Ohio Medical and Surgical Journal* 4 (November 1851): 112-116.

McIntyre, Charles. "The Percentage of College-Bred Men in the Medical Profession." *Medical Record* 22 (December 16, 1882): 681-684.

McNaughton, James. "Address Delivered before the Medical Society of the State of New York, February 8th, 1837." *American Journal of the Medical Sciences* 20 (August 1837): 469-475.

Miles, Mason M. "Medical Reform." *Chicago Medical Times* 13 (September 1881): 265-267.

Millasich, Vincent. "Eclecticism and Its Origin." *California Eclectic Medical Journal* 6 (December 1913): 299-301.

Osler, William. "The License to Practice." *Transactions of the Medical and Chirurgical Faculty of the State of Maryland 1889* (1889): 70-82.

Paine, Martyn. "A Lecture on the Improvement of Medical Education in the United States." *New York Journal of Medicine* 1 (November 1843): 367-378.

Parsons, James R., Jr. "Preliminary Education, Professional Training and Practice in New York." *Journal of the American Medical Association* 26 (June 13, 1896): 1149-1152.

Pritchett, Henry S. "The Classification of Medical Schools." *Association of American Medical Colleges Proceedings, 1915* (1915): 11-29.

———. "The Obligations of the University to Medical Education." *AMA Bulletin* 5 (January 15, 1910): 289-299.

Purrington, William A. "Manslaughter, Christian Science, and the Law." *Medical Record* 54 (November 26, 1898): 757-761.

Rauch, John H. "Address on State Medicine." *Journal of the American Medical Association* 6 (June 12, 1886): 645-652.

Reynolds, Dudley S. "The Present Status of the Medical Profession." *Journal of the American Medical Association* 20 (June 3, 1893): 618-619.

Rodman, J. S. "Impressions of Medical Teaching Gained from Ten Years' Experience with National Board Examinations." *Association of American Medical Colleges Proceedings, 1925* (1925): 70-75.

Savage, G. C. "Medical Education in the South." *Bulletin of the American Academy of Medicine* 4 (October 1899): 358-375.

Secondary Sources

Books

Anderson, Fannie. *Doctors Under Three Flags.* Detroit, 1951.

Aub, Joseph C., and Hapgood, Ruth K. *Pioneer in Modern Medicine: David Linn Edsall of Harvard.* Cambridge, Massachusetts, 1970.

Bailyn, Bernard. *Education in the Forming of American Society.* Chapel Hill, 1960.

Beall, Otho T., and Shryock, Richard H. *Cotton Mather: First Significant Figure in American Medicine.* Baltimore, 1954.

Bell, Whitfield J., Jr. *John Morgan: Continental Doctor,* Philadelphia, 1965.

Billroth, Theodor. *The Medical Sciences in the German Universities.* New York, 1924.

Binger, Carl. *Revolutionary Doctor.* New York, 1966.

Blanton, Wyndham. *Medicine in Virginia in the 17th Century.* Richmond, 1930.

Blauch, Lloyd E., ed. *Education for the Professions.* Washington, D.C., 1955.

Bond, Earl D. *Dr. Kirkbride and His Mental Hospital.* Philadelphia, 1947.

Bonner, Thomas N. *American Doctors and German Universities.* Lincoln, Nebraska, 1963.

Carson, Joseph. *History of the Medical Department of the University of Pennsylvania.* Philadelphia, 1869.

Cary, John. *Joseph Warren: Physician, Politician, Patriot.* Urbana, Illinois, 1961.

Cassedy, James H. *Charles V. Chapin and the Public Health Movement.* Cambridge, Massachusetts, 1962.

Chapin, William A. R. *History of the University of Vermont College of Medicine.* Burlington, 1951.

Chesney, Alan M. *The Johns Hopkins Hospital and the Johns Hopkins University School of Medicine: A Chronicle.* Baltimore, 1943.

Churchill, Edward D., ed. *To Work in the Vineyard of Surgery: Reminiscences of J. Collins Warren.* Cambridge, Massachusetts, 1958.

Cordell, Eugene F. *Historical Sketches of the University of Maryland School of Medicine*. Baltimore, 1891.

Corner, Betsy, and Booth, C. C. *Chain of Friendship: Selected Letters of Dr. John Fothergill of London, 1735-1780*. Cambridge, Massachusetts, 1971.

Corner, George W. *Two Centuries of Medicine: A History of the School of Medicine, University of Pennsylvania*. Philadelphia, 1965.

Cowen, David L. *Medical Education: The Queen's-Rutgers Experience*. New Brunswick, New Jersey, 1966.

———. *Medicine and Health in New Jersey*. Princeton, 1964.

Cremin, Lawrence A. *American Education: The Colonial Experience*. New York, 1970.

Crowe, Samuel James. *Halsted of Johns Hopkins*. Springfield, Illinois, 1957.

Cushing, Harvey. *Life of Sir William Osler*. Philadelphia and London, 1922.

Danforth, I. N. *Life of Nathan Smith Davis*. Chicago, 1907.

Duffy, John. *Epidemics in Colonial America*. Baton Rouge, Louisiana, 1953.

———. *A History of Public Health in New York City, 1625-1866*. New York, 1968.

———., ed. *Rudolph Matas History of Medicine in Louisiana*. Baton Rouge, Louisiana, 1962.

Felter, Harvey W. *History of the Eclectic Medical Institute*. Cincinnati, 1902.

Fishbein, Morris. *History of the American Medical Association*. Philadelphia and London, 1947.

Flexner, Abraham. *Henry S. Pritchett: A Biography*. New York, 1943.

Fulton, John F. *Harvey Cushing: A Biography*. Springfield, Illinois, 1946.

Gibson, James E. *Dr. Bodo Otto and the Medical Background of the American Revolution*. Springfield, Illinois, 1937.

Godfrey, E. L. B. *History of the Medical Profession of Camden County*. Philadelphia, 1896.

Goodman, Nathan S. *Benjamin Rush*. Philadelphia, 1934.

Hanawalt, Leslie L. *A Place of Light: History of Wayne State University*. Detroit, 1968.

Harrington, Thomas F. *The Harvard Medical School*. New York and Chicago, 1903.

Hindle, Brooke. *The Pursuit of Science in Revolutionary America*. Chapel Hill, North Carolina, 1956.

Horine, Emmet Field. *Biographical Sketch and Guide to the Writings of Charles Caldwell, M. D*. Brooks, Kentucky, 1960.

———. *Daniel Drake*. Philadelphia, 1961.

Kaufman, Martin, *Homeopathy in America: Rise and Fall of a Medical Heresy.* Baltimore and London, 1971.

Kelly, Howard A. *Cyclopedia of American Medical Biography.* Philadelphia and London, 1912.

Kett, Joseph. *The Formation of the American Medical Profession.* New Haven and London, 1968.

King, Lester S. *The Medical World of the Eighteenth Century.* Chicago, 1958.

Konold, Donald E. *History of American Medical Ethics, 1847-1912.* Madison, Wisconsin, 1962.

Langstaff, John Brett. *Doctor Bard of Hyde Park.* New York, 1942.

Mims, Edward. *Chancellor Kirkland of Vanderbilt.* Nashville, 1940.

Morse, John T. *Life and Letters of Oliver Wendell Holmes.* Boston and New York, 1897.

National Board of Medical Examiners. *Quarter of a Century of Progress.* Philadelphia, 1940.

Norwood, William F. *Medical Education in the United States Before the Civil War.* Philadelphia, 1944.

Puschmann, Theodor. *A History of Medical Education.* New York, 1966.

Reed, Alfred Z. *Training for the Public Profession of the Law.* New York, 1921.

Riznik, Barnes. *Medicine in New England, 1790-1840.* Sturbridge, Massachusetts, 1963.

Schachner, August, *Ephraim McDowell.* Philadelphia and London, 1921.

Schafer, Henry B. *The American Medical Profession, 1783-1850.* New York, 1936.

Shryock, Richard H. *The Development of Modern Medicine.* New York, 1947.

⸻. *Medical Licensing in America, 1650-1965.* Baltimore, 1967.

⸻. *Medicine and Society in America: 1660-1860.* Ithaca, New York, 1962.

Stookey, Byron, *A History of Colonial Medical Education in the Province of New York, with Its Subsequent Development, 1767-1830.* Springfield, Illinois, 1962.

Thoms, Herbert. *Jared Eliot.* 1967.

Thorpe, Francis Newton. *William Pepper, M.D., LL.D.* Philadelphia, 1904.

Waite, Frederick. *The First Medical College in Vermont: Castleton, 1818-1862.* Montpelier, 1949.

Warren, Charles. *History of the American Bar.* 1913.

Warren, Edward. *Life of John Collins Warren.* Boston, 1860.
———. *Life of John Warren, M.D.* Boston, 1874.
Wilder, Alexander. *History of Medicine.* New Sharon, Maine, 1901.

Articles

Atwater, Edward. "The Medical Profession in a New Society: Rochester, New York (1811-1860)." *Bulletin of the History of Medicine* 47 (May-June 1973): 221-235.
Bailyn, Bernard. "Communications and Trade: The Atlantic in the Seventeenth Century." *Journal of Economic History* 13 (1953): 378-387.
Bell, Whitfield J., Jr., "The Medical Institution of Yale College, 1810-1885." *Yale Journal of Biology and Medicine* 33 (December 1960): 169-183.
———. "A Portrait of the Colonial Physician." *Bulletin of the History of Medicine* 44 (November-December 1970): 497-517.
———. "John Morgan." *Bulletin of the History of Medicine* 22 (September-October 1948): 543-561.
———. "Medical Students and Their Examiners in Eighteenth Century America." *Transactions and Studies of the College of Physicians of Philadelphia,* 4th ser. 21 (June 1953): 14-24.
Blake, John. "Diseases and Medical Practice in Colonial America." *International Record of Medicine* 171 (June 1958): 350-363.
Bonner, Thomas N. "Dr. Nathan Smith Davis and the Growth of Chicago Medicine, 1850-1900." *Bulletin of the History of Medicine* 26 (July-August 1952): 360-374.
Bryan, Charles S. "Bloodletting in American Medicine, 1830-1892." *Bulletin of the History of Medicine* 38 (November-December 1964): 516-529.
Burwell, C. Sidney. "Medicine as a Social Instrument: Medical Education in the Twentieth Century." *New England Journal of Medicine* 244 (May 3, 1951): 673-684.
Cordell, Eugene F. "Our Alma Mater in 1807." *Maryland Medical Journal* 7 (October 1, 1880): 251-255.
Corner, Betsy C. "Early Medical Ecuation in Western New York, Geneva and Rochester Areas, 1827-1872." *New York State Journal of Medicine* 55 (November 1, 1955): 3156-3164.
Corner, George W. "Beginnings of Medical Education in Philadelphia, 1765-1776." *Journal of the American Medical Association* 194 (November 15, 1965): 719-721.
Doolen, Richard M. "The Founding of the University of Michigan Hospital:

An Innovation in Medical Education." *Journal of Medical Education* 39 (January 1964): 50-57.

Fitz, Reginald. "The Surprising Career of Peter La Terriere, Bachelor in Medicine." *Annals of Medical History,* 3d ser. 3 (September 1941): 395-417.

Fleming, Donald. "The Full-Time Controversy." *Journal of Medical Education* 30 (July 1955): 398-406.

Fox, Claire G. "Dr. Heber Chase: *The Medical Student's Guide." Bulletin of the History of Medicine* 42 (September-October 1968): 462-469.

Halstead, Frank G. "A First-Hand Account of a Treatment by Thomsonian Medicine in the 1830's." *Bulletin of the History of Medicine* 10 (December 1941): 680-687.

Heaton, Claude. "Medicine in New York During the English Colonial Period." *Bulletin of the History of Medicine* 17 (January 1945): 9-37.

Holt, Anna C. "A Medical Student in Boston, 1825-26." *Harvard Library Bulletin* 6 (1952): 176-192, 358-375.

Hudson, Robert P. "Abraham Flexner in Perspective." *Bulletin of the History of Medicine* 46 (November-December 1972): 545-561.

Jarcho, Saul. "Medical Education in the United States, 1910-1956." *Journal of the Mt. Sinai Hospital* 26 (1959): 339-385.

Jones, Russell M. "American Doctors and the Parisian Medical World, 1830-1840." *Bulletin of the History of Medicine* 47 (January-February 1973): 40-65 (March-April 1973): 177-204.

Jordan, Philip D. "The Secret Six, An Inquiry into the Basic Materia Medica of the Thomsonian System of Botanic Medicine." *Ohio State Archaeological and Historical Quarterly* 52 (October-December 1943): 347-355.

Kampmeier, Otto F. "Nathan Smith Davis, 1817-1904." *Journal of Medical Education* 34 (May 1959): 496-508.

Kaufman, Martin. "American Medical Diploma Mills." *Bulletin of the Tulane Medical Faculty* 26 (February 1967): 53-57.

Lawson, Hampden C. "The Early Medical Schools of Kentucky." *Bulletin of the History of Medicine* 24 (March-April 1950): 168-175.

Means, William J. "The History, Aims, and Objects of the Association of American Medical Colleges." *Proceedings of the Association of American Medical Colleges, 1919* (1919): 5-12.

Miller, Genevieve. "European Influences in Colonial Medicine." *Ciba Symposia* 8 (January 1947): 511-521.

―――. "Medical Apprenticeship in the American Colonies." *Ciba Symposia* 8 (January 1947): 502-510.

————. "Medical Education in the American Colonies." *Journal of Medical Education* 31 (February 1956): 82-94.

————. "Medical Schools in the Colonies." *Ciba Symposia* 8 (January 1947): 522-532.

Munger, Donna Bingham. "Robert Brookings and the Flexner Report." *Journal of the History of Medicine* 23 (October 1968): 356-371.

Norwood, William F. "American Medical Education from the Revolutionary War to the Civil War." *Journal of Medical Education* 32 (June 1957): 433-444.

————. "The Mainstream of American Medical Education, 1765-1965." *Annals of the New York Academy of Sciences* 128 (September 27, 1965): 463-472.

Numbers, Ronald L. "The Making of an Eclectic Physician: Joseph M. McElhinney and the Eclectic Medical Institute of Cincinnati." *Bulletin of the History of Medicine* 47 (March-April 1973): 155-166.

Olch, Peter D. "The Morgan-Shippen Controversy." *Review of Surgery* 22 (January-February 1965): 1-8.

Postell, William D. "Medical Education and Medical Schools in Colonial America." *International Record of Medicine* 171 (June 1958): 364-370.

Rogers, Fred B. "Nicholas Romayne, 1756-1817: Stormy Petrel of American Medical Education." *Journal of Medical Education* 35 (March 1960): 258-263.

————. "William Pepper, 1843-1898." *Journal of Medical Education* 34 (September 1959): 885-889.

Shryock, Richard H. "The Influence of the Johns Hopkins University on American Medical Education." *Journal of Medical Education* 31 (April 1956): 226-235.

Simmer, Hans H. "Principles and Problems of Medical Undergraduate Education in Germany during the Nineteenth and Early Twentieth Centuries." In C. D. O'Malley, ed. *The History of Medical Education.* Berkeley, Los Angeles, and London, 1970, pp. 173-200.

Smiley, Dean F. "History of the Association of American Medical Colleges, 1876-1956." *Journal of Medical Education* 32 (July 1957): 512-525.

Soutter, Lamar. "Medical Education and the University, 1901-1968." *New England Journal of Medicine* 279 (August 8, 1968): 294-299.

Steiner, Walter R. "Some Distinguished American Medical Students of Pierre-Charles-Alexander Louis of Paris." *Bulletin of the History of Medicine* 7 (1939): 783-793.

Stookey, Byron. "America's Two Colonial Medical Schools." *Bulletin of the New York Academy of Medicine* 40 (April 1964): 269-284.

————. "Origins of the First National Medical Convention: 1826-1846."

Journal of the American Medical Association 177 (July 15, 1961): 123-130.

Thomson, Elizabeth H. "Thomas Bond, 1713-84." *Journal of Medical Education* 33 (1958): 614-624.

Waite, Frederick C. "American Sectarian Medical Colleges before the Civil War." *Bulletin of the History of Medicine* 19 (February 1946): 148-166.

————. "Birth of the First Independent Proprietary Medical School in New England, at Castleton, Vermont, in 1818." *Annals of Medical History,* n.s. 7 (May 1935): 242-252.

————. "Medical Degrees Conferred in the American Colonies and in the United States in the Eighteenth Century." *Annals of Medical History,* n.s. 9 (July 1937): 315-320.

Waring, Joseph I. "The Influence of Benjamin Rush on the Practice of Bleeding in South Carolina." *Bulletin of the History of Medicine* 35 (May-June 1961): 230-237.

Weiskotten, Herman G. "Nicholas Romayne: Pioneer in Medical Education in the United States." *New York State Journal of Medicine* 66 (August 15, 1966): 2158-2177.

Womack, Nathan A. "The Evolution of the National Board of Medical Examiners." *Journal of the American Medical Association* 192 (June 7, 1965): 817-823.

Young, James Harvey. "American Medical Quackery in the Age of the Common Man." *Mississippi Valley Historical Review* 47 (1960-1961): 579-593.

Index

Castleton Medical College, 41, 45, 89
Chaillé, Stanford, 114, 122
Chalmers, Lionel, 8
Channing, Walter, 50
Chaplin, James P., 81, 114, 122
Chapman, Nathaniel, 50-51, 100
Chattanooga Medical College, 171
Cheselden, William, 10, 13, 14
Chicago Medical College, 113, 118, 127-28, 155
Chicago Medical Journal and Examiner, 138-39
Chicago, University of, 174. *See also* Rush Medical College
Christian Science, 146
Cincinnati College, 84, 98
Cincinnati, University of, 124
Civil War, 107, 158, 166
Clapp, Rev. Theodore, 61
Cleveland Medical College, 42-43, 99
Clinical instruction: AMA proposals on, 106; changing image of the hospital in, 133; in colonial period, 9-10, 14, 21-22, 24; after Flexner report, 179; in France and America, 100-102; at Geneva Medical College, 42; at Johns Hopkins, 148-150; at Medical College of Ohio, 49
Clossy, Samuel, 8, 23
Coale, Samuel, 27
Cock, Thomas, 90, 95-96
Cocke, James, 38
Colden, Cadwalader, 8
College of Physicians and Surgeons (Chicago), 169
College of Physicians and Surgeons (New York), 69, 94, 135; early years of, 36-38; evaluation of, 88;
reform at, 102, 127; and American Medical College Association, 137-39
College of Physicians and Surgeons of the Western District of New York (Fairfield), 36, 41
Columbia Law School, 166
Columbia University, 37, 177. *See also* College of Physicians and Surgeons (New York)
Colwell, Nathan P., 161, 164-67, 177-79
Commercial Hospital and Lunatic Asylum, 44
Condie, D. Francis, 106
Connecticut, license laws in, 122
Connecticut State Medical Society, 79
Connor, Leartus, 135, 137-39
Cooke, John E., 44, 50, 60-61
Cooper, Sir Astley, 38
Cordell, Eugene F., 155
Cornell Medical School, 152, 177
Couper, James, 90
Coxe, John Redman, 50
Crosby, Dixi, 106
Cullen, John, 89-90
Cullen, William, 8-9, 14, 22, 28, 57-58
Currey, R. C., 104-105
Curriculum: at College of Philadelphia, 20-23; graded, 127-28, 136-38, 148-51; post-Flexner, 179; proposed, 85, 94, 110
Cushing, Erastus, 42
Cushing, Harvey, 176
Cutler, Manasseh, 65

Danforth, Dr., 24-25

ABOUT THE AUTHOR

Martin Kaufman is associate professor of history at Westfield State College, Massachusetts.   He earned his A.B. at Boston University in 1962, his M.A. at the University of Pittsburgh in 1963, and his Ph.D. at Tulane University in 1969.

Dr. Kaufman's area of special interest is American social history and much of his research has focused on the history of American medicine and public health in America. His book *Homeopathy in America: Rise and Fall of a Medical Heresy* was published in 1971. He is currently at work on a dictionary of American medical history to be published by Greenwood Press, for which he is editor-in-chief.